Praise for *Mastering Herbalism*

"Presents rational advice on growing herbs, levelheaded chapters on herbs for longevity and herbs for love potions. One of the strongest points is the consumer-oriented listing of where to buy or order herbs in the U.S. and the United Kingdom. . . . Paul Huson is able to draw on the best of all possible worlds, what the Druids and the ancient cults of the Middle East knew and what the Anglo-Saxons called 'wortcunning,' or herbal magic, plus the bare bones measurements of modern science." — *Boston Globe*

"This 'must' book for witches includes a list of suppliers and a helpful bibliography." —*Detroit Free Press*

"A provocative account that will drive you to experiment and explore. Offers something to every reader." —*Baton Rouge Advocate*

"So with the aid of just one book, you can be healthy, quiet, or hilarious; make friends and influence people; grow your own perfumes; gain a reputation as a garden planner; and smell clean, without TV commercials." —*Nashville Banner*

"Tells you everything you always wanted to know regarding the secret power of herbs." —*El Paso Times*

"The author traces herbs in history and lists easily available herbs, which, he believes, can prolong life, cure diseases, improve cooking, make perfumes and incense, and possibly even make the heart grow fonder!" —*Los Angeles Herald Examiner*

"Extremely well organized with the essential information on using herbs medicinally, to cook with, to make perfumes, lotions, etc." —*Chattanooga Times*

T0307015

MASTERING

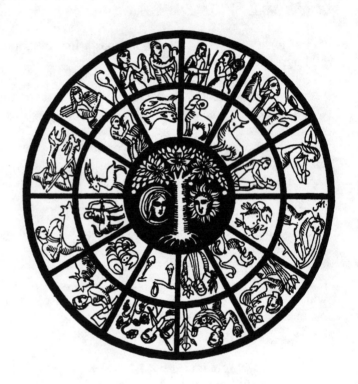

MADISON BOOKS
Lanham • New York • Oxford

HERBALISM

A PRACTICAL GUIDE

THE AGRICULTURAL YEAR

JANUARY: *With this fyre I warm my hand*
FEBRUARY: *With this spade I digge my land*
MARCH: *Here I cut my Vine spring*
APRIL: *Here I hear the birds sing*
MAY: *I am as fresh as bird on bough*
JUNE: *Corn is weeded well enough*
JULY: *With this sithe my grasse I mowe*
AUGUST: *Here I cut my corne full lowe*
SEPTEMBER: *With this flaile I earne my bread*
OCTOBER: *Here I sowe my wheats so red*
NOVEMBER: *With this axe I kill my swine*
DECEMBER: *And here I brew both ale and wine.*
—from *Ram's Little Dodoen,*
herbal of 1606

PAUL HUSON   *Illustrated by the Author*

Copyright © 1974, 2001 by Paul Huson
First Madison Books edition 2001

Designed by David Miller

Published by Madison Books
4501 Forbes Boulevard, Suite 200
Lanham, Maryland 20706

10 Thornbury Road
Plymouth PL6 7PP, United Kingdom

Distributed by National Book Network

Library of Congress Cataloging-in-Publication Data
Huson, Paul.
    Mastering herbalism : a practical guide / Paul Huson.— 1st Madison Books ed.
      p. cm.
    Originally published: New York : Stein and Day, 1974.
    "This Madison Books paperback edition of Mastering herbalism is an unabridged republication of the edition first published . . . in 1974, with the exception of an updated chapter nine ("Where to buy your herbs")."
    Includes bibliographical references and index.
    ISBN 1-56833-181-9 (pbk.: alk. paper)
    1. Herbs. 2. Herbs— Folklore. 3. Cookery (Herbs) I. Title.

GT5164 .H87 2001
635'.7— dc21   2001018324

⊖™ The paper used in this publication meets the minimum requirements of American National Standard for Information Sciences— Permanence of Paper for Printed Library Materials, ANSI/NISO Z39.48–1992.
Manufactured in the United States of America.

For Griselda

FOREWORD

IF YOU ARE IN THE HABIT of browsing through plant stores, as I am, you may on occasion find yourself confronted by an intriguing array of pots containing mysterious little herbs. The name tags they display, if there are any, are usually bluntly noncommittal and uncommunicative. "Wormwood—medicinal" is a typical one. Your interest may flare for an instant, but then die just as swiftly. How on earth would you use it anyway, just supposing it did actually grow in your planter or backyard?

What is the "herb mystique"? Just what can you do with those enigmatic little plants? Well, you can eat them and brew them into health-giving teas, or bathe in them and smoke them, or pound them up and plaster them all over your face and body; or you can grow them and dry them and perfume yourself and your friends with them; or you can wash your hair in them. More than that, you can follow age-old traditions and if you are talented in that direction, even cast spells with them. And last, but by no means least, you can live to a ripe old age by means of them.

And that, in a nutshell, is what this book is all about. My aim throughout is practicality. It is all very well to read an old herbal which says (if indeed it says anything about dosages), "Take ten minims of this and one fluid drachm of that," but where does that leave you with your pot of basil in the kitchen window? Basically all you will need for my kind of herbalism will be a couple of covered enamel or Pyrex pans, a cup, a small pestle and mortar (obtainable from any kitchen-supply store), a wineglass, a tablespoon, a teaspoon, and, if you're feeling adventurous, a teapot—regular kitchen

7

equipment, in fact. Plus, of course, your usual gardening tools if you feel like growing your own. If you don't, never mind. Herbs are among the easiest things to get by mail. They qualify for third-class mailing privileges, and there are any number of excellent mail-order companies you can get them from. Chapter 9 lists a fairly extensive selection of these.

CONTENTS

MASTERING
HERBALISM

Introduction: HERBS IN HISTORY

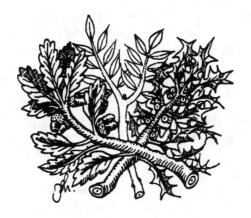

Of all the trees that grow so fair
Old England to adorn
Greater are none beneath the Sun
Than Oak and Ash, and Thorn.[1]

WHEN YOU EAT AN HERB, YOU partake of history. Plants were here before we were, and if they survive the current ecological crisis they will probably still be here after we have gone. They are patient and enduring, and remarkably persistent, and the lifetimes of the greatest among them—the "Oak and Ash, and Thorn"—are numbered in multiples of our own. The lesser species—mere wayside herbs —"anything green that grew out of the mould," as the same poet humorously refers to them, have for centuries been valued by the wise more highly than jewels or precious metals. And for good reason.

In their blossoms, seeds, leaves, and roots are locked the secrets of life and death, powers healing or harmful depending on how they are used. Herbs have been used from time immemorial as medicines, tonics, body beautifiers, mind stimulants; as aphrodisiacs, perfumes, and smoke-makers. They can impart rare and special flavor to food, yield alcoholic beverages, and, of course, produce altered states of consciousness, for many are psychoactive agents. Many of these, unlike marijuana and peyote, are still quite

[1] Rudyard Kipling, *Puck of Pook's Hill.*

legally obtainable. Even immortality can be attained by the use of herbs—or so people once said. Stranger still, some are beginning to say so again, if by immortality you mean cell regeneration.

Then there is the fascinating lore of the occult powers of herbs. Witchery has always made extensive use of them, often for their powerful chemical properties, but equally often for properties of which the average person is not so well aware. Many recognize the existence of extrasensory perception in people, but what is not so well known is that this same mysterious power of communication extends into the plant kingdom too. There is more to the so-called green thumb than mere tender loving care, and the Oak and Ash, and Thorn hold more secrets than merely chemical constituents like tannin, fraxin, and ilicin, as we shall see in later chapters.

This is a beginner's herbal, and my aim throughout has been practicality rather than erudition. The history of the subject is, of course, endlessly fascinating, and could fill an encyclopedia. For the sake of conciseness, however, I have restricted it for the most part to this first, introductory chapter. A precise knowledge of where an herb came from and by whom it was introduced is by no means mandatory for the lay herbalist. Herb lore has traditionally been handed down from master to apprentice, at first simply by word of mouth. What was passed down was the knowledge of which herb worked and which did not. Only with the advent of printing did a more scholarly approach become possible.

THE ANCIENT WORLD

Herbalism has been practiced for at least five thousand years, probably more. Its origins, like those of many bodies of traditional lore, are rooted far back in prehistory. At first man took his nourishment where and how he could, hunting deer and bison and gathering edible plants haphazardly. He appears to have settled down and begun raising plants and animals methodically only during the New Stone Age, after the northern icecaps had melted, transforming the wastes of Europe into temperate forest regions. Between 4000 and 3000 B.C. the invention of the potter's wheel, the wheel itself, bricks for building, and, most important of all, the discovery of copper and bronze did more to speed civilization than anything else has done. Prior to that he used stone implements and animal horns for his tools and weapons.

Around 3000 B.C. men began moving westward through Europe and crossing the ever-widening newly melted polar waters which now divided the mainland from the British Isles, bringing with them their knowledge of cattle breeding and wheat farming. At about the same time the pharaoh Narmer was unifying Upper and Lower Egypt and founding the first recorded pharaonic dynasty. In Mesopotamia the Sumerians were inventing their cuneiform writing. Herbs were undoubtedly being used. However, it was in the Far East that our first detailed reference to herbs was made a few hundred years later, in what was an advanced civilization even in those early days. Shen-Nung, the "Red Emperor"—so called on account of the "fiery" quality of his personality—used himself as a guinea pig to study the effects of various herbs upon the human constitution. He came to the conclusion that the ginseng plant was the king of all herbs and a genuine promoter of longevity, and even today the Chinese think of it as just that. Shen-Nung's own long life seems to have given eloquent support to his observations, for he died at the ripe old age of 123!

Fifteen hundred years later, in 1500 B.C., the Egyptian pharaoh Thothmes III dispatched an expedition to Syria in search of new and useful medicinal plants, among other things. Reliefs of some of the plants it returned with can be seen to this day carved upon the walls of Thothmes' own temple in Karnak. Among them are quite recognizable sunflowers, irises, pomegranates, lotuses, and arum-lilies, all of them once highly valued botanical medicines. We know from the books of the Old Testament that a large variety of herbs and spices besides these were also raised in ancient Mesopotamia. The prophet Jeremiah, for instance, alludes to balm of Gilead, a rare aromatic gum which the historian Josephus tells us was presented as a gift to the resplendent King Solomon by none other than the Queen of Sheba. The Song of Solomon mentions camphor, spikenard, saffron, calamus, cinnamon, frankincense, myrrh, and aloes—all still considered valuable items in the herbal pharmacopoeia.

It was the versatile and innovative Greeks, however, who made the first serious attempt in the West to systematize their herbal lore in writing. Between 500 and 400 B.C. a number of lists of herbs began to appear, all of them attributed to the famous physician Hippocrates, the Father of Medicine. They catalogue and describe between three and four hundred useful plants. Although their actual authorship is highly debatable, Hippocrates' name helped to earn them lasting respect down the centuries. The lists were shortly improved upon around 400 B.C. by a botanist from Eubeoia, Diocles of Carystus, whose book is now recognized as the first complete Western herbal. Soon after Hippocrates died, the ships of Alexander the Great began returning from their conquest of the East laden with plunder. Herbs and exotic spices were included among the other treasures. Mangrove, cotton, and euphorbium made their appearance in the Western world, alongside such now-familiar spices as cinnamon and saffron. Theophrastus of Eresus, like Alexander a pupil of Aristotle (and so devoted a gardener that he willed his body to be buried in one of his own flowerbeds to feed his flowers), capitalized upon this influx of new Oriental herb lore in his *History of Plants*, which he wrote in about 300 B.C. Besides providing a handy encyclopedia of useful plants, common and exotic, Theophrastus also reveals tantalizing glimpses of the dark workings of the Rhizotomists, a fraternity of herbalists who wove their lore into a semireligious cult and practiced magical rituals strongly reminiscent of those of the Druids, the mysterious oak priests of ancient Britain. The Rhizotomists continued as a coherent cult well into the Christian era, and a considerable amount of Saxon "wortcunning" and medieval herbal witchcraft is demonstrably derived from their practices. The earth is worshiped as a mother; she must be prayed to and placated when herbs are plucked; the herbs themselves are addressed before being gathered; the stars and the moon must be observed to find the right astrological moment when the herbs will be most powerful. We shall take a closer look at some of the fascinating lore derived from these beliefs in Chapter 6.

Drawings of herbs did not begin to appear in herbals until the first century B.C. Crateuas, a member of the Rhizotomists and attendant upon the Parthian king Mithridates VI, wrote a botanical treatise containing sketches of aristolochia, which numbers among its immediate family the birthwort, the snake-root, and

Asarum europeum, an herb once used by Egyptian sorcerers like those contested by Moses to stupefy serpents.

Only when the herbal came West once more, did it get arranged in alphabetical order. The herbal of Pamphilus of Rome provides our first example of this in the first century A.D. In the same century the chronicler (he can hardly be called a botanist or scientist) Pliny the Elder gathered together a vast quantity of old beliefs and herbal lore, the tattered remnants of many fading religious cults, in Books 12–19 of his *Natural History,* an encyclopedic work which enormously influenced early medieval thinking. More scientific was the attitude displayed by Galen, a Greek physician to the Roman emperor Marcus Aurelius, who insists in his great treatise on medicine of the same period that the wise physician should learn to recognize herbs for himself rather than leave himself wide open to being deceived by the itinerant Roman *herbarii,* or herb peddlers. Galen also tells us that Roman emperors of his day were in the habit of employing herbalists from Sicily, Crete and Africa, and thought nothing of sending as far afield in quest of their herbs as Syria, Egypt, India, Spain, and Gaul.

Probably the most influential work in the field of early medicine, and undoubtedly so in the area of herbs, was the work of a humble army doctor to the Roman legions (although some say he was personal physician to Antony and Cleopatra). His name was Pedanius Dioscorides, and he lived around 50 A.D. His *De Materia Medica* provided the main source for all other Western and Eastern herbals thereafter, and for that matter, still continues to do so. It was translated into Persian, Hebrew, Arabic, Provençal, Anglo-Saxon, and other languages, and it marked the emergence of herbalism as a definite, demonstrable discipline as opposed to simply a collection of travelers' tales and arcane beliefs like those of the Rhizotomists.

THE DARK AGES

The wise physicians of the Arabian empire were not slow to recognize the value of Dioscorides' monumental work. Neither were those of Byzantium. And as is the way with all influential works, imitations began appearing. Around 400 A.D. the Latin *Herbarium of Apuleius the Platonist* boldly and unashamedly plagiarized Dioscorides, blithely noting that its supposed author had sat at the feet of none other than the centaur Chiron, that great legendary herbalist of Greek myth. Ironically, the Apuleius, not Dioscorides, was destined to become the prototype for most medieval herbals: it was written in Latin, which made it accessible to many, whereas the Greek of the original Dioscorides was available to only the most educated. Dioscorides was finally translated into Latin in the sixth century A.D. at the instigation of Cassiodorus, the powerful chancellor to Theodoric the Great, king of the Ostrogoths and later emperor of Rome. The Latin Dioscorides provides amazingly methodical listings of herbs under Latin, Greek, Punic, Tuscan, Egyptian, Syrian, Gallic, Spanish, and even biblical names. Early copies also contain pagan occult formulas: the earth is again invoked as "Holy Mother Earth"; circles are required to be drawn with a knife around the herb under consideration and so on, although in later versions these elements are purged to make place for more pious Christian prayers.

The tenth-century Anglo-Saxon *Leech-book of Bald and Cild* ("Bald owns this book; Cild is the one he told to write it," the introduction explains helpfully) drew upon the now accessible herb lore of Dioscorides, but combined it with such Saxon folklore as that given in the famous *Lacnunga*, an eleventh-century medical spell-book containing the epic incantation now known as the "Nine Herbs Charm." Bald and Cild also apparently obtained special royal permission to make use of certain Eastern herbal prescriptions in the possession of King Alfred the Great.

By the eleventh century, Dioscorides and Apuleius had become required reading for the students at the first schools of medicine in Europe, the Benedictine monastery of Monte Cassino, and the community of healers at Salerno. What makes the school of Salerno really remarkable, and indeed sets it apart from all other educational institutions of the time, was the fact that it admitted women as well as men, a generally quite unheard of practice.

THE MIDDLE AGES

Throughout the Middle Ages, most monasteries followed the example of Monte Cassino and studied herbalism. Dispensing Christian charity, which included healing the sick, was after all one of their primary duties. Each monastery owned its private herbary, or herb garden, and of course every library had its copies of Apuleius and Dioscorides, now lavishly illustrated in color and gold leaf. To this day, monastery ruins still frequently contain old medicinal herbs growing among the weeds.

The first printed herbal did not appear until 1484, about forty years after the printing process was invented. It was an Apuleius, and it was printed in Rome. A landmark, it provided the next step toward making herbal knowledge generally available to the public.

THE SIXTEENTH AND SEVENTEENTH CENTURIES

A German physician born in 1493, Theophrastus Bombastus, otherwise known as Paracelsus, complicated herbalism's evolution as a science with his "Doctrine of Signatures." Simply stated, it claimed that every plant was "signed" or associated by a mysterious spiritual bond to a particular disease. The clue to which disease this was could be found in the shape, color, scent, or even habitat of the herb itself. For instance eyebright, *(Euphrasia officinalis)*, whose flowers hold a resemblance to bright eyes, was considered (and for that matter still is) a good remedy for sore eyes and ophthalmia. Lungwort *(Sticta pulmonaria)*, on the other hand, whose spotted leaves were thought to resemble lungs, was held efficacious for bronchial complaints. Often, as in the case of these two plants, the results obtainable from their use really do coincide with their "signature"; whether through the workings of some mysterious law or just by coincidence it is impossible to say. From an orthodox medical point of view, the Doctrine of Signatures is of course outrageous nonsense. Yet who knows but that what we dismiss as coincidence today will not turn out to be the workings of some long-suspected but hitherto unproved principle in nature? Certainly Paul Kammerer, Carl G. Jung, and lately Arthur Koestler would seem to think so.

John Gerard's *Herbal* of 1597 proved to be the next great turning point in herbal history. Columbus had introduced America to the Western world in 1492, and in the same way that Alexander's expedition had benefited early herbalism, so did that of Columbus. Gerard's famous herbal exhibited to Europe's fascinated gaze many exotic and hitherto unknown plants from "the New Lande called America," among which were the potato, the tomato (called by him "the Apple of Love"), and tobacco.

In 1551 "the Father of British Botany," William Turner, dean of Wells Cathedral, published his *Nieuwe Herball*. Going on the very sensible assumption that the customary practice of writing herbals in Latin had not only outlived its usefulness but now even constituted an actual danger to the half-educated reader, who might be tempted to rush in and try an herb without fully comprehending the accompanying instructions, Turner wrote his herbal in a common tongue: English. Thus the herbal's passage from the libraries of the privileged to the hands of the public was finally assured. Herbalism under the Tudors became a common pursuit. All large households incorporated herbaries or "paradise gardens," as they now came to be called, in their rambling estates. However, the herbs that grew in them now were used as much for their fragrance as for their healing powers. Perfumed pomanders, clove-stuck oranges were carried by wealthy Elizabethans to combat the appalling stenches they were confronted with every day. Sweet bags and sachets filled with lavender, rosemary, and bergamot also served to help. Many householders continued to strew their halls with sweet-smelling herbs after the fashion of the Middle Ages. Even small Tudor cottages could be expected to possess gardens containing the above-mentioned plants in addition to others equally fragrant: balm, thyme, costmary, spearmint, and, of course, the ever-present English rose. Rural doctors began to cultivate their own herbs rather than rely upon those they found growing wild in the surrounding countryside. In 1573 Thomas Tusser's *Five Hundred Pointes of Good Husbandrie* introduced some of the age-old horticultural lore of planting by moon and tide to the reading public. Tusser's homey snippets of rhymed astrological advice quickly found an audience among farmers only too glad to at last have an almanac which set down in print some of the old, traditional country wisdom they had received from their grandparents and always relied upon.

The herbalist Nicholas Culpeper, whose name is perhaps the most well known, successfully combined astrology with herbalism after the manner of ancients some seventy-three years later in his famous *Complete Herbal* (1653). Astrology had become popular fad in Culpeper's day, so he had a ready-made audience.

"Such as are astrologers (and indeed none else are fit to make physicians) such I advise," he states unequivocally in the section dealing with culling and drying herbs. Many present-day herbalists consider Culpeper's book a great step back into the Middle Ages for herbalism. Others see it as a sign of the times, a revolt against the steadily growing spirit of rationalism, and a harking back to romantic, mythical roots. It certainly reintroduces an element of poetry to herbalism which was fast disappearing with the advance of seventeenth-century science. The only other herbal that had introduced astrological lore was a 1550 edition of the popular *Banckes's Herbal*, written in 1525 by one Richard Banckes, about whom we know nothing.

Culpeper's romanticism and the remnants of Paracelsus' doctrines notwithstanding, the seventeenth century produced a host of eminent scientifically inclined herbalists. John Parkinson, the herbalist royal to Charles I, wrote two encyclopedic volumes of botanical lore, the *Theatrum Botanicum* and *Paradisi in Sole Paradisus Terrestris*. Parkinson grew herbs in his own herb garden at Holborn, which he referred to lovingly in his books as his "Garden of Pleasure." Popular herbals were also written by Matthias de L'Obel, who gave his name to the pretty blue lobelia plant (still used in asthma cures), and William Coys, a botanist responsible for introducing the spiky ornamental yucca plant to England. John Goodyer was another big name in herbals; he translated Dioscorides into English in 1655. Sir John Salusbury made his name by compiling the first Welsh-language herbal. But already the art of the herbalist was giving place to the science of the apothecary. The paradise gardens and herbaries of old were fast being replaced by more practical-sounding physick gardens.

THE EIGHTEENTH AND NINETEENTH CENTURIES

Academic interest in herbalism all but died with the advent of the eighteenth and nineteenth centuries, although in rural districts in Britain, Europe, and the United States herbal medicine continued to be popular and useful. C. F. Millspaugh's *American Medicinal Plants*, written in 1887 and still a classic in the field, supplemented and enlarged the European herbal pharmacopoeia with a wealth of native American plants. One notable exception to the general drift toward chemically derived drugs was the theory and practice of homeopathy devised by the German physician Samuel Hahnemann (1755–1843). Homeopathy contained echoes of the teachings of Paracelsus, but made use of minute amounts of vegetable drugs, which are, of course, the active ingredients in many of the more potent herbs. Hahnemann believed that diseases could be cured by applying herbal remedies which would produce, in a healthy person, symptoms similar to the ailments of the patient, a development of the old Doctrine of Signatures into modern terms. As with present-day vaccines, just "a hair of the dog": obviously a concept not to be dismissed.

HERBALISM TODAY

During the twentieth century, official interest in herbs revived in a dramatic and quite unforeseen manner, strangely enough due to the outbreak of the two world wars. Britain and Europe twice found themselves cut off from their Oriental and American drug supplies, and thus forced to fall back on their own indigenous resources: herbs. During World War II the Soviet Union also took up large-scale herb farming, as did Italy. Germany and France had always had plentiful herbs of their own, growing wild. In Britain the Ministry of Supply began to organize methodical herb cultivation; schoolchildren were induced to go on forays for medicinal herbs and vitamin C-rich rose hips; gardeners were urged to reserve a patch in their yards for useful drug-producing plants as well as for table vegetables.

The last of the great herbals was published in the interim between the two world wars. Hilda Leyel (who wrote under the name Mrs. C. F. Leyel) had founded the Society of Herbalists Ltd. in 1927. Committed to the cause of herbalism and convinced of its overlooked usefulness, she successfully courted publicity by housing her new company in a storefront in Baker Street, Sherlock Holmes's old stamping ground. The shop became an immediate success. People were indeed receptive to herbalism once more. Four years later, in 1931, Mrs. Leyel edited and published the famous and monumental *Modern Herbal,* using as its basis a series of herb pamphlets written by a Buckinghamshire herbalist, Mrs. M. Grieve, but supplementing them with her own American and European researches. Leyel and Grieve's remarkable book is now regarded as the standard, most complete herbal encyclopedia in the English language.

Interest in herbs has grown steadily over the past forty years. During the last ten it has, of course, received a considerable boost from publication of books like Aldous Huxley's *Doors of Perception* and the interest they have sparked in botanical psychoactive agents such as cannabis and peyote. But the wave of involvement in plants and herbs that is sweeping the Western world is far more general, and cannot be said to be limited to those who are simply exploring the plant world for its potential psychoactive properties. Yellow air, dying rivers and seas, and the ever-increasing destruction of wildlife are only the more obvious parts of the price we pay for the gifts of a modern technology. Hardly surprisingly, ecology has become more than just a public byword of the seventies. Now people are discovering that there is something talismanic about plants: they are green, exuberant, and natural. Above all they are natural. Whether you eat them or just keep them in your home to look at is almost beside the point. It is their "naturalness" which counts: to grow them is to make an affirmation of life itself in a desert of artifice and garbage. Of course, this flight from technology is not new to history, but the scale of today's version of it is. Men of the last century who advocated a return to nature, like Blake, Wordsworth, Coleridge, and Thoreau, were isolated cases in their day and age. Or maybe they were simply the vanguard of ours. For undoubtedly large numbers of men and women today are finally catching on to Gandhi's notion that there is something that sets living things apart from the artificial and merely useful. Of course, with herbs you can have it both ways, for here are plants that satisfy both requirements, the old pragmatic one and the new vitalist one. Even when you buy them dried, they still share in the aliveness, although at one stage removed. The world is, after all, a totality, with all its parts interacting. In a sense all lives are one Life; all parts however small, plant or man, are integral to the Whole, for the energy which spins the atom also moves the galaxy. Plants and herbs were among the first offspring of Mother Earth, first upon the evolutionary ladder.

As we have seen, the man-plant communion has been a long one, spanning many thousands of years of history, only five of which are recorded, but undoubtedly stretching back to the day of man's first discovery of plants as a food source. In all those millennia herbs have lost none of their power. They worked for Shen-Nung five thousand years ago and they worked for Dioscorides. They continued to work for Gerard, Turner, and Parkinson, and today half the wonder drugs of our modern pharmacopoeia are either derived from them or were discovered first in their fibers. Maybe they can work for us too.

> Of herbys now I
> Will you telle by and by . . .

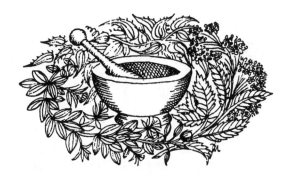

1

HERBS TO STAY HEALTHY WITH

UP UNTIL FAIRLY RECENTLY, THE nearer to town you got in Europe or the United States, the less likely you were to run across herbal medicine. This is not the case any more. Of course, herbs have always been looked upon favorably by country folk and still are, but today they are being rediscovered by the city-dweller. This is partly due to the advent of the ubiquitous health-food store and mail-order company, and partly to the fact that the urbanite is beginning to appreciate herbs' real values, two of which are outstanding: 1) Herbs seem to possess a mysterious power of helping you to stay healthy which commercial brands of tonics and vitamins frequently lack; and 2) As medicines, herbs often do the job for common complaints just as effectively (if not more so) as many of the commercial pills and nostrums on the pharmacy counter, and are generally far less expensive. Not that the lay herbalist can ever replace the qualified doctor when it comes to any ailment more serious than colds, sprains, sleeplessness, indigestion, and so on; although I should also add that there are people who swear that herbal medicine has produced results for them where orthodox treatment has failed lamentably.

If herbalism does have any claim to superiority over regular medicine—and the controversy still rages—it lies in the difference between organically derived drugs and chemically derived ones.

Committed herbalists believe that the herb in its unprocessed, natural state contains, alongside its active principle or alkaloid, organic and uncounterfeitable food which provides both a nourishment and a stimulus for the exhausted cells of the human body. This food consists of a highly complex natural synthesis of organically derived salts, vitamins, and nutrients which in commercial drug products are usually considered extraneous and therefore omitted. Chemists will counter this with the argument that the amount of alkaloid contained within a herbal dose cannot be accurately measured owing to fluctuating regional variations, and so on. This is obviously true. But practiced herbalists are not stupid, and if they know their job they always take these factors into consideration. Balance in the composition of the herb blend is a matter of the highest importance. Herbal medicine at its most refined is not a hit-or-miss affair but a genuine science acquired after much study and practice.

It is not my intention in this chapter to woo the reader away from his family doctor by giving him a selection of cure-alls. The training required for the competent practice of herbal medicine is just as exacting as that of any other therapeutic discipline. Many of the more potent herbs contain powerful vegetable drugs which can be extremely dangerous if improperly administered. Herbs like foxglove and belladonna, these are the "big guns" of herbalism and we shall not be concerning ourselves with them in this chapter. There also exist a large number of benevolent, easy to grow, and no less useful herbs which are to an herbalist what his basics are to a cook. He knows them as "simples," and the use of them as the art of "simpling."

THE ART OF SIMPLING

Most of the herbs I shall describe here have been used for many centuries for a wide spectrum of ailments. The uses I ascribe to them are the most popular or the most up to date. All the herbs are easy to grow or obtain, many of them from your local grocery, nearly all from your local health-food store; definitely all from the efficient herb mail-order houses listed at the back of this book.

Try experimenting with these herbs singly at first as simples, noting the effect they have (or don't have) on you, for not everyone reacts to an herb in the same way. Build up your collection as you go along.

STORING HERBS

Herbs you buy in groceries will often come in glass jars of their own, but those you order by mail will almost invariably be sent in plastic or waxed-paper bags. The mail-order variety will, incidentally, be half the price, sometimes less, of those bought in a store. You may keep them in their plastic bags, of course—this way they squash into any convenient corner or drawer—or you can bottle them yourself. Most stores dealing with fancy kitchenware handle a line of suitable herb jars, often in racks. We shall be dealing with that and related matters in greater detail in Chapter 8. For now it will be sufficient to say that the ideal herb jar is one made of opaque material, such as ceramic or colored glass (to prevent the herbs from spoiling in the sunlight), with a screw top, ground-glass stopper, or tight cork to prevent moisture from entering. If you do settle for clear-glass containers, make sure your shelves are not in direct sunlight. A closable herb cabinet is ideal, and can be purchased from kitchenware stores or easily constructed. Always label your jars in type, or a good, clear hand, preferably using an indelible ink. The reason for this is obvious: one dried herb looks remarkably like another. Use self-adhesive labels, for the plain gummed variety will often peel off the jar when it dries.

LATIN NAMES

Although it may seem an unnecessary bore at first, it really is a good idea to familiarize yourself with the Latin names of your herbs. The reason is simple: common herb names change depending on what country or region you are in; Latin names do not. For instance, there are two plants that go by the name of marigold. One of them is supposed to help you get well and the other is not.

GROWING YOUR OWN

If you decide to grow herbs of your own, so much the better. Herbs freshly gathered and dried are, generally speaking, preferable in two respects to shop-bought ones: though the active principles of store-bought varieties remain intact, their nutritive and aromatic qualities are often depleted because of overlong storage. With mail-order herbs the chances of freshness are much better, but they still cannot compete with the home-grown variety. Chapters 8 and 9 will deal with various methods of indoor and outdoor cultivation and drying, or ordering by mail.

HOW TO ADMINISTER HERBS

Most of the following herbs do not need to be ingested directly, but can be taken in the form of an *infusion*, the herbalist's term for a tea made by pouring boiling water over the dried herb. When an herb takes time to yield its essence (usually when it comes in bark or root form), either it is administered in a powdered form or a *decoction* is made from it, which simply means that it is boiled in water in a covered pot for a given period of time. The strained liquid is then administered.

Many of the herbs in this chapter are *aromatics*, which means simply that they smell and taste good. These are the ones also used in cooking—thyme and peppermint, for instance. They make the most palatable infusions, and may be drunk simply with the addition of a little sugar or, better still, honey. To those herbs not remarkable for their taste, however, it is customary among herbalists to add a hint of aromatic, often a spice, which not only makes up for the taste deficiency but also aids the digestion. Always plan on having one or two aromatics on hand for this purpose, even if you do not maintain a regular culinary spice rack. Here is a list of some of the most easily available and useful ones:

USEFUL AROMATICS

Allspice	Cardamom	Coriander	Orange peel
Anise	Cinnamon	Ginger	Vanilla bean
Caraway	Clove	Lemon peel	

Make sure you don't overdo your spice, though. One part aromatic to 4 parts other herbs (by weight) is more than enough. Experiment to find your favorite flavor and aroma. Cinnamon, clove, and lemon and orange peel are often selected.

HERBAL MEDICINES

Elementary medicines can be blended from a selection of herbs by means of a formula such as the following:

> 3 parts active (medicinally potent) herb or herbs
> 1 part aromatic, or spice
> 1 part demulcent herb

Simply select one or more herbs suitable for aiding the condition in question. Let us say you intend to compose a mildly sedative tea to drink before going to bed at night: you might choose lime flowers, camomile, and lemon verbena as your active herbs. Take 1 part each of these by weight, totaling 3 parts in all. Add to these 1 part aromatic. (Here you might choose orange or lemon peel or a blend of both.) Finally add 1 more part of a *demulcent* herb, such as coltsfoot. A demulcent is an herb that possesses soothing, mucilaginous qualities which help to allay any internal irritation.

USEFUL DEMULCENTS

Arrowroot	Licorice root	Sago root
Borage	Marsh-mallow leaves	Sassafras pith
Coltsfoot	and root	Slippery elm bark
Comfrey root	Oatmeal	Solomon's-seal root

Coltsfoot, comfrey, and marsh mallow can be grown in your own herb garden or purchased from your nearest health-food store or mail-order herb company.

Generally speaking, for a simple herb tea like the one mentioned above, 1 teaspoon herbs to 1 cup boiling water is a good rule of thumb. Use honey or sugar to flavor them if you wish; honey is better for you, however. Where powerful herbs such as valerian are used, special instructions will be given.

Two last things to observe: First, when you make an herb blend, make sure the mixture is uniform before you try infusing any. Every herb counts, remember. Second, do not try to keep your infusions over long periods. Make them fresh each time. Unless you keep them in a refrigerator, add alcohol, or turn them into a syrup, they will go "off" like any other vegetable matter and begin fermenting. If you want a real herbal beer or wine, see Chapter 2.

Traditional Cures

Here are some of the simpler herbal cures. Where a Latin name is given in parentheses, the herb in question, though a useful one, does not appear in the following pages, either because it comes from a tree, or because it is difficult or unsuitable to grow in an herb garden, or because of the large quantity needed (for instance, parsley seed), which can best be obtained in bulk from a commercial source.

Symbols: * Infuse 1 teaspoon herb to 1 cup boiling water. † Decoct 1 teaspoon herb in 1 cup boiling water. ‡ Powerful herb; use only with caution as prescribed by pharmacist.

Symbol	Meaning	Symbol	Meaning
℔·J·	pound	Σ	sugar
ANA	equal amounts		alcohol
℥·J·	ounce		honey
ʒ·J·	dram		mix
℈·J·	scruple		boil
P·J·	pinch	℞	take
	pint		distill
	still		filter
	retort		essence
	receiver	P	powder
	vinegar		compose

HERBALISTS' SYMBOLS

BLOOD PURIFIERS. Agrimony. Burdock root (*Arctium lappa*).[†]
Yarrow.

BURNS. Balm of Gilead. Comfrey. Elder. Yarrow.

COLDS AND FEVERS. Agrimony. Angelica root. Balm. Boneset
(*Eupatorium perfoliatum*, to be drunk in a cold infusion).
Camomile. Catnip. Elder flowers * (*Sambucus nigra*). Fenugreek *
(*Trigonella foenum graecum*). Feverfew. Horehound. Hyssop. Pen-
nyroyal. Peppermint. Sage. Spearmint. Thyme. Verbena. Worm-
wood. Yarrow.

CONGESTION. Coltsfoot. Comfrey root. Horehound. Mullein.

CONSTIPATION. Butternut root (*Juglans cinerea*). Dandelion.
Cascara sagrada.[‡] Senna.[‡]

COUGHS. Agrimony. Angelica root. Coltsfoot. Comfrey. Elecampane * (*Inula helenium*). Feverfew. Garlic. Horehound. Hyssop.
Marsh mallow. Nettle leaves * (*Urtica dioica*, or *Urens*). Red clover
tops * (*Trifolium pratense*). Speedwell * (*Veronica officinalis*).
Thyme. Vervain. Yerba santa (*Eriodictyon glutinosum*).

CUTS AND ABRASIONS. Burnet. Cranesbill (*Geranium maculatum*). Garlic. Marigold. Marsh mallow. Meadowsweet. Plantain.
Southernwood. Thyme. Valerian. Woodruff.

DIARRHEA. Borage. Cinquefoil. Comfrey. Marjoram. Marsh
mallow. Nettle leaves.* Plantain.

EMMENAGOGUES. Blue cohosh (*Caulophyllum thalictroides*).[‡]
Motherwort. Parsley seed * (*Apium petroselinum*). Pennyroyal.
Rue. Sage. Southernwood. Tansy. Wintergreen leaves * (*Gaultheria
procumbens*).

FLATULENCE. Angelica root. Bergamot. Catnip. Marjoram. Pennyroyal.

HEADACHE. Basil. Camomile. Lavender. Rosemary. Thyme.
Wood betony * (*Betonica officinalis*).

HEMORRHAGE. Red rosebuds.*

HICCUPS. Dill. Fennel. Juniper berry. Spearmint.

INDIGESTION. Camomile. Dill. Garlic. Marjoram. Pennyroyal.
Peppermint. Savory. Spearmint. Thyme. Verbena. Woodruff.

KIDNEY ACTION, TO PROMOTE. Angelica root. Borage. Dandelion.[†]
Garlic. Fennel. Feverfew. Meadowsweet. Parsley root [†] and leaves.

MOUTHWASH AND GARGLE. Agrimony. Cinquefoil. Fenugreek.*
Goldenrod. Raspberry leaves * (*Rubus idaeus*). Sage. Thyme.

NAUSEA. Basil. Bergamot. Golden seal (*Hydrastis canadensis*).‡ Marjoram. Pennyroyal. Peppermint. Spearmint.

PERSPIRATION, TO PROMOTE. Angelica root. Balm. Burnet. Camomile. Catnip. Elder flowers. Garlic. Hyssop. Lime (linden) flowers * (*Tilia europoea* or *vulgaris*). Pennyroyal. Thyme. Yarrow.

POULTICES. Comfrey root.† Garlic. Marsh mallow. Plantain. Sage. Thyme.

RHEUMATISM. Angelica root. Basil. Buckbean * (*Menyanthes trifoliata*). Hyssop.

SEDATIVES. Bugleweed.* Camomile. Catnip. Hops. Lady's slipper (*Cypripedium pubescens*; use ½ teaspoon herb to 1 cup boiling water). Lime, or linden, flowers.* Motherwort. Mullein. Primrose. Skullcap. Valerian. Verbena.

SPOTS AND PIMPLES. Agrimony. Speedwell * (*Veronica officinalis*).

SPRAINS. Comfrey root.† Marsh mallow. Sage. Wormwood.

STIMULANTS. Anise seeds * (*Pimpinella anisum*). Cinnamon. Cloves. Coffee beans. Elecampane.* Feverfew. Garlic. Ginger root.† Goldenrod. Hawthorn * (*Crataegus oxyacantha*). Hyssop. Lavender. Lovage. Marigold. Marjoram. Pennyroyal. Peppermint. Rosemary. Rue. Sage. Savory. Southernwood. Spearmint. Tea * (*Theaceae*). Vervain. Woodruff. Wormwood. Yarrow. Yerba maté * (*Ilex paraguayensis*).

STOMACH CRAMPS. Bergamot. Burdock leaves. Camomile. Coltsfoot. Comfrey root. Fenugreek. Marsh mallow. Meadowsweet. Peppermint. Sage. Thyme.

TEETHING TROUBLE. Clove. Peppermint. Yarrow.

TONIC, BODY-BUILDING. Alfalfa * (*Medicago sativa*).

TONICS. Agrimony. Buckbean. Burnet. Catnip. Centaury * (*Erythrae centaurium*). Camomile. Coltsfoot. Dandelion. Feverfew. Lovage. Marjoram. Meadowsweet. Motherwort. Nettle leaves.* Rosemary. Sage. Sarsaparilla † (*Smilax sarsaparilla*). Sassafras * (*Sassafras officinale*). Southernwood. Thyme. Vervain. Wormwood.

VERTIGO. Primrose.

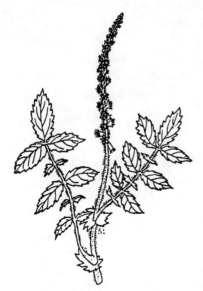

AGRIMONY
Agrimonia eupatoria

OTHER NAMES. Church steeples. Cocklebur. Sticklewort. Philanthropos. Common agrimony.

HABITAT. In its wild state, agrimony can be found growing extensively throughout Europe, Canada, and the United States. A hardy perennial, its natural habitat is woods and fields, but it takes to cultivation easily. Its one- to two-foot branchy stems are covered with a fine, silky down and terminate in spikes of cream-colored flowers. Both the flowers and the notched leaves give off a faint characteristic lemony scent when crushed. After the flowers fade they give place to tiny clinging "burrs" which will quickly adhere to your clothing if you brush by the plant in a hedgerow. For garden growing, give the herb sun or partial sun and regular watering, and plant from seed or propagate by root division in spring or fall. Gather the herb in summer while the flowers are in bloom.

PROPERTIES. Agrimony contains tannin and a volatile, essential oil. Like most simples, the uses to which it is put are remarkably varied. The English use it to make a delicious "spring" or "diet" drink for purifying the blood. It is considered especially useful as a tonic for aiding recovery from winter colds and fevers. As agrimony also possesses an astringent action, it is frequently used as an herbal mouthwash and gargle ingredient, and is applied externally in the form of a lotion to minor sores and ulcers. Mrs. M. Grieve recommended a strong decoction of it to cure sores, blemishes, and pimples.

HOW TO USE IT.

Agrimony tea, a Gentle Blood Purifier

Infuse 1 teaspoon dried agrimony root, leaves, or flowers in 1 cup of boiling water for 15 minutes. Strain and flavor with honey and a little licorice root if desired. Take up to 1 cup per day.

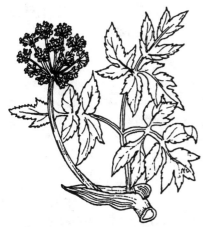

ANGELICA
Angelica archangelica

OTHER NAMES. *Archangelica officinalis.* Garden angelica. Archangel. Masterwort.

HABITAT. Once considered a sovereign remedy against witchcraft and the Powers of Darkness, angelica was originally a native of Syria, but now has been naturalized in Europe and the United States. It grows up to 6 feet in height and, as it likes a shady position and moist soil, you should plant it toward the rear of your herb garden. It comes from the same family as fennel and parsley, and possesses the same characteristic hollow, fluted stems of all these Umbelliferae. Its highly serrated leaves grow in bunches of three, and it exudes a sin-like fragrance when bruised. It is a hardy biennial herb (that is, it takes two years to reach maturity) and is extremely easy to grow from seed, root cutting, or seedling. However, if you plant from seed, make absolutely sure the seeds are freshly harvested, as they lose their vitality very quickly.

Only the seeds and roots are used in medicines; the latter should be carefully washed and dried on a wire rack first (see Chapter 8).

PROPERTIES. The herb contains, among other things, a volatile aromatic oil, sugar, valeric acid, angelic acid, and a resin known as angelicin. Herbalists use it to aid in the elimination of toxins, the recovery from rheumatism and colds, urinary complaints, and colic.

HOW TO USE IT.

Root Dosage

Infuse 1 ounce dried chopped root in 1 pint boiling water for ½ hour in a covered container. Drink 2 tablespoons of the liquid, flavored with honey if you wish, 3 or 4 times daily.

Seed Dosage

Infuse 1 teaspoon seed in 1 cup boiling water; cover. Allow to stand until cool; strain and drink 1 to 2 cups cold a day, again flavored with honey if desired.

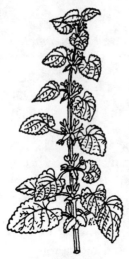

BALM
Melissa officinalis

OTHER NAMES. Sweet balm. Lemon balm. Garden balm. Melissa.

HABITAT. The name Melissa comes from the Greek meaning bee, which indicates this herb's long-recognized fine bee-attracting capacity. For this reason it was an old favorite for planting around hives. John Gerard mentions that in the sixteenth century the leaves were even rubbed upon the hives in an effort to keep the bees happy. The plant possesses a short root and a squarish stem (when cut sectionally) with joint pairs of toothed, heart-shaped, or oval leaves sprouting on either side of it. Both the leaves and the creamy yellow flowers give off a strong lemony smell when crushed. Though the leaves and stems die off each year, the root is perennial, which makes it a good choice for your herb garden. It will thrive in any type of soil, and can be grown from seed, seedling, root division in spring or fall, or cutting (if you are clever). Like most of the simples in this chapter, it requires the absolute minimum of attention: just make sure it has enough water, gets weeded from time to time, and has its straggling dead wood cut back in the fall. (As a treat for it you may also stir the earth between its roots once or twice a year.)

PROPERTIES. Balm has been used from time immemorial as a wound dressing, for it is rich in ozone and therefore strongly antiputrescent. It also makes a flavorful and mildly sedative tea to aid in opening the pores to reduce fevers produced by Flu or chest colds.

HOW TO USE IT.

Lemon-balm Tea

Infuse 2 teaspoons dried herb in 1 covered cup boiling water for 15 minutes. (Or 1 ounce herb to 1 pint boiling water if a larger quantity is required.) Strain, and flavor with sugar or honey and a twist of lemon, if desired, before drinking.

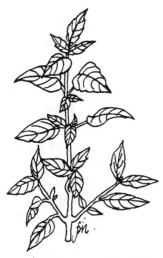

BASIL
Ocimum basilicum

OTHER NAMES. St. Josephswort. Sweet basil.

HABITAT. Once native to India and Persia only, and still a sacred herb to the Hindus, basil is an annual plant much used now in Mediterranean cookery. It grows up to 2 feet in height, and its one drawback is that it must be raised from seed or seedling each year. It likes a rich moist soil with plenty of sun. You can buy various types of basil besides the "sweet" variety, the other most popular being "bush" basil. All possess the same properties, however.

The herb grows with a square stem in section; smooth, slightly toothed, oval leaves, which give off a strong clove fragrance when crushed; and white, pink, or red whorls of flowers which nestle in the axils of the leaves (where the leaf joins the stem).

PROPERTIES. Basil contains an aromatic and volatile camphor-bearing oil which gives it its marvelous clovelike fragrance and accounts for its use in cooking, potpourris, and perfumery. A delicious tea can also be prepared from the leaves which is thought to allay mild nervous tension headaches and nausea.

HOW TO USE IT.

Basil Tea

Infuse 1 teaspoon dried herb in 1 covered cup boiling water, strain, and flavor with honey if desired. Up to 1 or 2 cups a day may be taken.

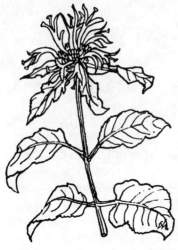

BERGAMOT
Monarda didyma

OTHER NAMES. Monarda. Scarlet monarda. Oswego tea. Bee balm. Red bee balm.

HABITAT. This prolific perennial herb bears delightful scarlet flowers beloved by bees for their nectar. Its hard, square, grooved stems grow up to 3 feet tall, and the rough, dark, paired leaves which branch off from them, when crushed, exude an exotic fragrance strongly reminiscent of bergamot oranges.

Bergamot is very easy to grow, preferring a light moist soil in either sun or shade. However, as with all the other mints, you will have to keep an eye on its roots to make sure they do not begin to strangle your other herbs. (Many gardeners plant mints in boxes or pots only for this very reason.) Such is the exuberance of the bergamot, you will probably be able to divide it every 3 years, keeping one clump and giving away the others to your friends.

PROPERTIES. Bergamot is a rich source of thymol, an aromatic antiseptic substance used extensively in modern medicine and dentistry. The chief value of the herb for the herbalist, however, is as an infusion to benefit an upset stomach, nausea, and vomiting.

HOW TO USE IT.

Bergamot Tea

Infuse 1 teaspoon dried bergamot in 1 covered cup boiling water for fifteen minutes. Strain and add honey to flavor.

BONESET
Eupatorium perfoliatum

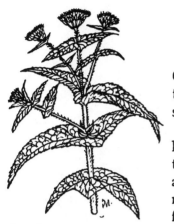

OTHER NAMES. Thoroughwort. Eupatorium. Ague weed. Crosswort. Indian sage.

HABITAT. Boneset grows wild in low-lying damp fields and meadows throughout the United States, although its seeds can be bought from nurseries specializing in herbs. An old favorite of the American Indians, no plant has been more extensively used in native American herbalism than this one. The Menominees, Iroquois, and Mohegans used it as a febrifuge; the Creeks as an anodyne; and the Alabamas as a stomachic. C. F. Millspaugh, the great nineteenth-century herbalist, wrote an account of how boneset cured a friend of his malarial fever which had hitherto resisted any other remedy, including quinine. Boneset is a slightly aromatic, perennial herb with a cylindrical downy stem which grows from 2 to 4 feet high, branching out at the top into flower stems. The finely serrated, tapering leaves grow opposite one another on the stem, joining one another in a curious and distinctive fashion at their bases and giving the impression of a leafy collar through which the stem pokes—hence the Latin name *perfoliatum*. Their texture is rough and wrinkled on the surface but downy underneath, with prominent veins running through them. The white flowers which appear in July to September grow in rounded tufts at the end of the flower stems. The herb should be planted in sun or light shade and given plenty of water.

PROPERTIES. The name boneset indicates its traditional use as an herb given, not as one might think, to assist the union of fractured bones, but rather to cure a virus once prevalent in the United States, commonly known as breakbone fever. Herbalists today know it as a gentle but powerful diaphoretic, stimulant, laxative, and febrifuge. It is taken as a warm infusion in moderate doses to combat muscular rheumatism, colds, and fevers. In larger doses it becomes a laxative and emetic. Cold doses are taken as a tonic.

HOW TO USE IT.

Mrs. Grieve advocates boneset as a specific for flu. She recommends 1 ounce of the dried herb infused in 1 pint boiling water. The patient, remaining in bed the whole time, should take 1 warm wineglass every half hour, up to 4 or 5 doses. As a tonic, 1 level teaspoon dried herb is infused for 30 minutes in 1 cup boiling water. The resultant liquor is strained and 1 teaspoon taken cold 3 to 6 times a day.

BORAGE
Borago officinalis

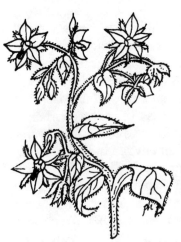

OTHER NAMES. Common bugloss. Burrage.

HABITAT. Originally a native of Aleppo, but now naturalized all over Europe and the United States, this pretty annual will grow from 1 to 3 feet in height. Its round stems are branched, hollow, and full of juice; its pointed oval leaves are dark or gray-green and wrinkled. The entire plant is covered with a bristly silvery-gray down, and its blue star-shaped flowers hang in leafy clusters from the end of the stems. It does well in poor soil in either sun or shade with medium watering, and will seed itself if allowed, although it can be grown from cuttings if desired.

PROPERTIES. Borage is rich in potassium, calcium, salt, and mucilage, and is therefore highly valued for its demulcent qualities. French herbalists use it to ease fevers, but in England and the United States it is administered for chest colds and kidney complaints.

HOW TO USE IT.

Borage Tea

Infuse 1 ounce dried leaves in 1 pint boiling water for 15 minutes. Strain and flavor with honey if desired. Take by the wineglass.

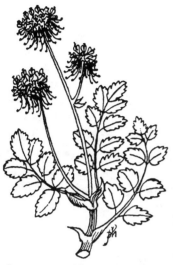

BURNET
Pimpinella saxifraga

OTHER NAMES. Italian burnet. Salad burnet. Burnet saxifrage. Italian pimpernel. *Pimpinella sanguisorba.*

HABITAT. Burnet was one of the favorite herbs of the Tudors, who used to plant it in narrow pathways with thyme and camomile so that when trodden on its fragrance would give additional enjoyment. But it has been used by herbalists since even earlier days: long before Culpeper prescribed it as an antidote to melancholy, Pliny mentions it as a useful herb. Originally a native of Europe, it was introduced to the United States by the first settlers, possibly the Pilgrim fathers themselves. The burnet is a perennial herb. Its rounded, toothed leaves grow in pairs upon their own stem, and its upright white or reddish flowers produce tiny, berrylike fruit. It will grow between 1 and 2 feet in height, and prefers a dryish, well-drained soil with plenty of sun. It will seed itself if it is allowed to, and you can produce extra plants by dividing its roots during the spring or fall.

PROPERTIES. Seventeenth-century herbalists like Nicholas Culpeper considered burnet to be an excellent cure for the blues. He advocated steeping 3 sprigs of the herb in a cup of wine, preferably claret, as a cordial to "quicken spirits, refresh and clear the heart, and drive away melancholy"! Most present-day herbalists, however, consider burnet more useful first as a diaphoretic, that is, an herb which induces perspiration to eliminate toxins; and secondly as an astringent for bathing small sores and abrasions.

HOW TO USE IT.

Burnet Tea

Infuse 1 teaspoon dried herb in 1 covered cup boiling water. Strain and flavor if desired, and drink up to 1 cup per day.

Astringent Lotion

Decoct in a covered vessel 1 handful dried herb in 1 pint boiling water for 15 minutes. Strain and allow to cool before using.

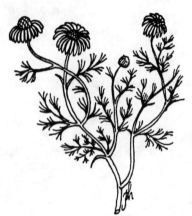

CAMOMILE
Anthemis nobilis

OTHER NAMES. Maythen. Manzanilla.

HABITAT. Once a favorite of Anglo-Saxon herbals, camomile was used like burnet during the Middle Ages and in the sixteenth century as a perfumed ground cover for the paths in the gardens of large houses. It is an evergreen perennial, and the more you tread on it—or so they say—the better it grows! Although generally a low, ground-hugging herb, it can grow up to 12 inches in height, especially when it sends up its long flower stems. The flowers themselves look like tiny white daisies with rayed petals and golden centers, and both they and the finely divided light-green leaves will give off a delicious vanillalike fragrance when you crush them. Give camomile as much sun as you can, but keep the soil moist at all times. You can sow the seeds in early spring or late fall, but it is much easier simply to plant snippets from the root runners of old plants, treading them into the ground well as you would with lawn sets. Because of its delicacy, you will have to weed your camomile by hand rather than hoe it.

PROPERTIES. Camomile contains, among other things, calcium, tannic acid, glucoside, and anthemic acid. It is used chiefly for aiding upset stomachs, as a tonic infusion, and as a gentle *nervine*. In older herbalists' language, this means simply a medicine that acts on the nerves—what today we would call a tranquilizer. It also happens to make a really delicious tea.

HOW TO USE IT.
Camomile Tea
Infuse 1 ounce dried blossoms for 15 minutes in 1 pint boiling water. For a single cup, infuse 1 teaspoon flowers in 1 cup boiling water. Strain and flavor with honey if desired.

Note: As the value of camomile rests chiefly in its volatile essential oil, always make sure the container in which you make your infusion is covered while in use, not an open cup.

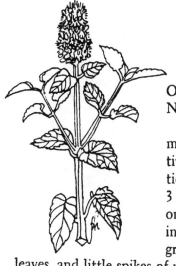

CATNIP
Nepeta cataria

OTHER NAMES. Catnep. Nep. Catmint. Nip.

HABITAT. Catnip belongs to the enormous family of mints and, like its relatives, possesses the same square (in section) stems and branches. Growing up to 3 feet in height, this rugged perennial, once a native of Europe and Asia but now introduced to the United States, bears grayish downy heart-shaped or oval leaves, and little spikes of whitish or pink flowers. It needs only a regular soil and hardly any watering in which to flourish but, like all the mints, will take over your garden if you give it half a chance. You can break up your clumps of catnip in spring or fall and throw out the older wood, or keep slips of root for planting elsewhere.

Cats, of course, are driven wild by the strange bitter fragrance of this herb, and will come from miles around to roll in it, although rats, not illogically one would think, are said to detest it.

PROPERTIES. Catnip is claimed to be stomachic (soothing to an upset stomach), tonic, and diaphoretic in effect. However, outweighing all other properties are its nervine qualities.

HOW TO USE IT.

Mild Sedative

Infuse in a covered pot 1 ounce dried catnip in 1 pint boiling water. Allow to cool, and strain. Flavor if desired. Adults: 2 tablespoons; children: 2 to 3 teaspoons.

For an Upset Stomach

Infuse 1 teaspoon herb in 1 covered cup boiling water. Up to 2 cups per day may be drunk.

Note: Catnip tea when drunk warm in large quantities can have an emetic effect on some people. Many herbalists advise letting it cool before using.

THREE TONIC CATNIP BLENDS

1. Mix together:

> 2 parts catnip
> 1 part motherwort
> 2 parts skullcap
> 1 part sage
> 2 parts camomile

Infuse 1 teaspoon blend in 1 covered cup of boiling water. Strain after 10 minutes and sweeten with honey if required. Drink 1 wine glassful 3 times a day and before going to bed.

2. Mix together:

> 1 part catnip
> 1 part camomile
> 1 part spearmint
> 1 part marjoram

Prepare as above.

3. Mix together:

> 2 parts catnip
> 1 part bruised celery seed
> 3 parts skullcap

Infuse 1 teaspoon in a covered cup of boiling water for 15 minutes, strain, and flavor with honey if required. Drink 1 lukewarm cup up to 4 times a day.

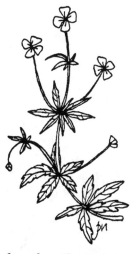

CINQUEFOIL
Potentilla reptans

OTHER NAMES. *Potentilla canadensis.* Five-finger grass. Five-leaf grass. Five fingers. Five-finger blossom. Sunkfield. Synkefoyle.

HABITAT. An old-time favorite of witches and sorcerers, probably on account of its roughly pentagram or hand-shaped leaf, this creeping herb will need to be watched lest it invade your herb garden and start choking the other plants. Its palmate, serrated leaves grow on stems ranging from 2 to 18 inches in length, off which branch small yellow flowers that close at night, each to its own stalk. Valued in herbal medicine since the time of Hippocrates and Dioscorides, the cinquefoil now grows all over Europe and the United States. It will do best in rich, well-watered soils.

PROPERTIES. Since Dioscorides' day, cinquefoil has been employed as a febrifuge—that is, a medicine with the property of abating or mitigating fever. Because of its astringent qualities, it is also used as a lotion for washing cuts and abrasions. Mrs. M. Grieve also recommends that the infusion be employed as a sore-throat gargle, and as a cure for diarrhea.

HOW TO USE IT.
Cinquefoil Infusion
Infuse 1 ounce dried herb in 1 pint boiling water. Cool and strain. Flavor with sugar or honey and take in wineglass doses if required for internal application.

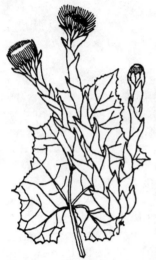

COLTSFOOT
Tussilago farfara

OTHER NAMES. Coughwort. Hallfoot. Horsehoof. Ass's foot. Foalswort. Field-hove. Bullsfoot. Donnhove. Horse-foot. Ginger root (U.S.). Filius ante pater.

HABITAT. Coltsfoot's old Latin country name, *filius ante pater* (son before father), is an indication of its growing habits. Its bright-yellow flowers appear some time before the long-stalked, hoof-shaped, serrated leaves, which are covered with woolly down when young but become smooth as they grow older. A native of both Europe and the United States, coltsfoot will flourish if you plant it in damp, clayey soil. The faintly aromatic dried leaves were once dipped in saltpeter and used as tinder before the invention of matches.

PROPERTIES. Coltsfoot contains a variety of medicinally useful elements. Notable among them are the minerals calcium, potassium, and sulphur. Vitamin C is also present, as are mucilage and tannin. The flowers contain a substance called phytosterol. Coltsfoot's uses are as varied as its constituents: Its mucilage makes it a handy demulcent and emollient; its mineral and vitamin content, a tonic. It is also a popular cough medicine.

HOW TO USE IT.

Coltsfoot Cough Decoction

Mrs. M. Grieve recommends letting 1 ounce dried coltsfoot leaves placed in 1 quart water boil down to 1 pint of liquid. The resultant liquor should be strained and sweetened with honey and 1 teacup taken as often as required. Less strong but needing less preparation is simple *Coltsfoot Tea:*

Steep 1 teaspoonful of the herb in 1 cup water for 30 minutes. Strain and flavor with honey. Take ½ cup 2 to 3 times daily and once before retiring.

COMFREY
Symphytum officinale

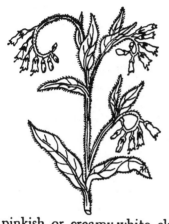

OTHER NAMES. Common comfrey. Healing herb. Blackwort. Knitbone. Knitback. Consound. Bruisewort. Slippery root. Boneset. Yalluc. Gum plant. Consolida. Ass ear. Wallwort.

HABITAT. Comfrey grows with a hollow, downy, angular stem up to 3 feet in height around ponds and in low-lying ditches. Its flowers hang in pinkish or creamy-white clusters, and its leaves have a pleasant medicinal smell about them. You may plant comfrey in any type of soil, but if you have a shaded area, especially under a tree, then choose that spot by preference. Propagation is usually accomplished by seed during the fall, or by root division. Water regularly, and keep the herb clear of weeds.

The name *officinale* indicates that a plant was once in the old monkish pharmacopoeia, and indeed comfrey is just such an old-time favorite.

PROPERTIES. Comfrey contains potassium, tannin, allantoin, and mucilage. In the Middle Ages its chief claim to fame, as its names "boneset" and "bruisewort" suggest, lay in its value as a poultice ingredient. Although it is still extensively used today for this—the entire fresh plant is beaten to a pulp and applied as a hot compress to the sprain or inflamed part—it is now also employed as an expectorant for coughs and colds and as a demulcent diarrhea decoction.

How TO USE IT.
Comfrey Bronchial Infusion

Infuse 1 ounce of the leaves in 1 pint boiling water. Let stand for ½ hour or longer. Strain, and flavor with honey if desired. Drink 1 to 2 cups per day. For a lesser amount, use 1 teaspoon herb to 1 cup boiling water.

Comfrey Diarrhea Decoction

Boil ½ ounce dried, crushed comfrey root in 1 quart water or milk. Take in wineglass doses as often as needed.

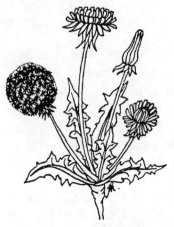

DANDELION
Taraxacum officinale

OTHER NAMES. Blow ball. Priest's crown. Cankerwort. Swine's snout.

HABITAT. You may not think you need or want this humble herb in your herb garden, for it grows practically everywhere, and is, of course, the bane of gardeners. Its thick, dark root is practically impossible to eradicate from lawns, where it delights to grow. However, despite its wretched garden reputation, the dandelion is famous and revered in the books of herbalists, and it is ironically just those long, tenacious roots which contain the major portion of its wealth of natural minerals and alkaloids! Its name means "lion's teeth," and if you look at its serrated leaves you will see how appropriate this is.

PROPERTIES. Dandelions contain calcium, magnesium, potassium, vitamins A and E, taraxacin, taraxacerin, inulin, gum, and gluten. The acrid milky juice in the stems is used in Derbyshire, England, to remove warts. The roots, which should be gathered in fall, winter, or spring, are tonic, diuretic, and laxative; the yellow flowers and leaves are tonic.

HOW TO USE IT.

Dandelion Tonic Tea

Infuse 1 ounce dried yellow flowers and leaves in 1 pint boiling water for 10 minutes. Strain and sweeten with honey. You may drink up to several glasses during the course of the day.

An Infusion for Biliousness

Infuse 1 heaping teaspoon chopped dried dandelion root in 1 cup boiling water for 30 minutes. Drink 1 or 2 cups daily.

An Old Remedy for Jaundice

Old-time herbalists used to employ the following decoction to aid in recovery from jaundice. As in the above recipe, dandelion is here employed for its traditionally beneficial effect on the liver. Take:

1 ounce dried, chopped dandelion root
½ ounce ginger root
½ ounce caraway seed
½ ounce cinnamon bark
¼ ounce senna leaves

Boil in 3 pints water until only 1½ pints remain. Strain the resultant liquid, add ½ pound sugar, and return to the boil. Skim, strain, and cool. Dose with frequent teaspoons.

DILL
Anethum graveolens

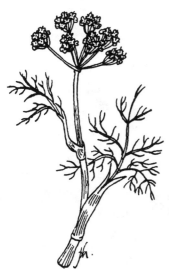

OTHER NAMES. *Fructus anethi.* Dill weed.

HABITAT. Once a hardy native of the Mediterranean lands and southern Russia, dill came west with the Romans, and later farther west with the American settlers. Its name derives from the Norse stem *dilla,* meaning "to lull." It was originally considered to be a good cure for insomnia, not so much for any sedative values it might possess, but rather on account of its digestive ones: it is, of course, a primary ingredient of babies' dill water. Possibly because of its soothing effects, it has always been held in high repute as a plant capable of putting evilly disposed night-riding witches and demons to flight.

Trefoil, vervain, John's wort, dill,
Hinder witches of their will!

says the old rune.

Dill will grow from 2 to 3 feet in height, and will produce an abundance of feathery leaves sprouting from bright-green upright stems topped by small umbrellalike tufts of yellow flowers. Because of its height, plant it toward the back of your herb garden, in full sun if you can manage it. Make sure it has good drainage, and if you intend to grow the herb from seed, sow it in March or April.

PROPERTIES. Dill contains two essential oils: limonene and carvone, which today make it valuable as a digestive aid, and a cure for hiccups.

HOW TO USE IT.

Dill Tea

Take 2 teaspoons dried dill seeds and leaves. Bruise them in a pestle and mortar, and infuse them, covered, in ½ pint boiling water. Strain when cool, and take 2 ounces every hour or two until the condition is alleviated.

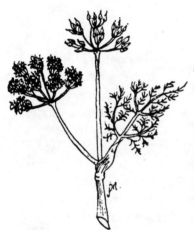

FENNEL
Foeniculum officinale

OTHER NAMES. Wild fennel. Sweet fennel. Large fennel. Fenkel.

HABITAT. Another ancient herb introduced to Western Europe by the Romans, fennel, like its close cousin dill, was also used extensively in both medicine and sorcery. Pliny mentions twenty-two remedies in connection with it, and it is one of the mysterious "nine herbs" in the eleventh-century Saxon charm of the same name.

Although its leaves die off every year, fennel possesses a thick perennial rootstock from which the smooth, shiny stems spring. Like dill and most other members of the Umbelliferae family, fennel's leaves are tiny and segmented, and its bright-gold flowers which appear in summer also have a similar umbrellalike structure. Unlike dill, however, which is more fastidious about its habitat, fennel will grow practically anywhere, ideally in a light, well-drained soil. But it does need plenty of sun. If sown early in April it may grow up to 5 feet in height by the end of the summer, so be careful where you place it in your garden.

PROPERTIES. When you crush the leaves and fruit of the fennel, you will become immediately aware of its strong, aniselike fragrance. Herbal fragrance of whatever kind is always a sure indication of the presence of essential oils. In fennel's case these are anethol (the same oil contained in anise) and fenchone. Fennel also contains traces of potassium, sodium, and sulphur.

On account of its essential oils, fennel's chief use in herbal medicines today is as gentle digestive stimulant, aromatic, and diuretic to promote kidney action.

How to use it.

Fennel Tea

Infuse 1 teaspoon dried, bruised fennel seeds and leaves in ½ pint boiling water. Cover and let cool, then strain, and flavor as required before taking.

Fennel Blend Digestive Tea

Mix equal parts of

Fennel seeds
Anise seeds
Coriander seeds
Caraway seeds

Bruise 1 teaspoon seeds, and prepare exactly as above, drinking cool or hot, as preferred.

FEVERFEW
Chrysanthemum parthenium

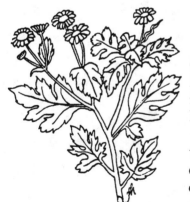

OTHER NAMES. Bachelor's buttons. *Pyrethrum parthenium.* Featherfew. Febrifuge plant. Featherfoil. Flirtwort.

HABITAT. Feverfew comes from the same family as the garden chrysanthemum. Its leaves, when crushed, give off a highly pungent odor which is said to be extremely offensive to bees and other insects. The leaves themselves are light green, sharply cut in shape, and covered with a silky down. They last through the winter. The flowers are numerous, small, white, and daisylike with flat yellow centers; the stems furrowed, hairy like the leaves, extending as high as 2 feet or more.

When grown from seed, feverfew should be sown in February or March and planted out in June. However, as in the case of chrysanthemums, root division or cuttings taken from the woody stems of old plants and inserted in the ground during the winter months are much easier to grow. Give the herb a reasonably moist soil in sun or partial shade.

PROPERTIES. Feverfew is used by herbalists as a tonic, a sedative, an aromatic, and a mild laxative.

HOW TO USE IT.

Tonic Tea

Infuse 1 ounce dried feverfew in 1 pint boiling water. Cover and let the infusion cool before straining. Drink in ½ teacup doses, flavored with honey if desired.

Mild Sedative

Infuse 1 ounce dried feverfew flowers in 1 pint boiling water as above. Drink *cool*, flavored with honey if desired.

For Colds and Fevers

Infuse 1 ounce dried feverfew flowers in one pint of boiling water. Drink *hot*, flavored with honey if desired.

GARLIC
Allium sativum

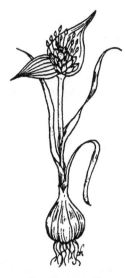

OTHER NAME. Poor man's treacle.

HABITAT. You may be surprised to find the garlic listed here, but it is actually one of the more important simples known to herbalists. Once a native of southwestern Siberia, the lowly garlic has now spread throughout Europe and the United States. Theophrastus of Eresus tells us the ancient Greeks used to place it at the crossroads as an offering to Hecate, the goddess of witchcraft and sorcery. Homer states that Ulysses owed his narrow escape from being changed into an animal by the enchantress Circe to the virtues of the garlic. Certainly Transylvanian vampires are rumored to be held at bay by its potency, as every horror-film buff knows. Curiously enough, recent scientific research has found in garlic a combination of antiseptic and mosquito repellent. In that the "touch of the vampire" was generally a dramatic synonym for plague or disease often brought on by the bite of mosquitoes, one is forced to wonder whether the old Romanians were really so misguided in their applications of the plant.

Garlic will flourish best in moist, sandy soil in a sunny position. The bulb is easy enough to obtain whole from your nearest grocery. (Make sure the head you buy has not dried out completely.) Simply divide it into its component cloves, and insert them in the soil about 2 inches deep. Keep them about 6 inches apart. If you plant them in spring, they should have produced five healthy plants, each with its own bulb, by August or September, at which time the long scallion-like leaves will have begun to die off. If you are lucky, you may even have had a pale, whitish flower or two.

PROPERTIES. Garlic contains an essential oil known as sulphide of allyl. The pungent smell of the herb is that of the sulphur contained in it. Herbalists use garlic for its diaphoretic (perspiration-producing) and diuretic (kidney-stimulating), properties.

It also comes in handy as an antiseptic, a cough medicine, and a stimulant. Because of the last attribute, garlic powder is pre-scribed in capsule form by some herbalists as a brain developer.

How TO USE IT.

Garlic Cough Syrup

Considered by many herbalists to be a sovereign remedy for bronchial complaints ranging from asthma to bronchitis.

Slice 1 pound fresh garlic bulbs and boil them until soft in 1 quart water, adding ½ ounce each of bruised fennel and caraway seed. Let this stand for 12 hours in a closely covered container before straining. Add to the resultant liquor an equal quantity of vinegar, bringing it back to the boil, and add enough sugar to make it into the consistency of a syrup. One spoonful of syrup may be taken each morning and whenever necessary.

Four Thieves Vinegar

A Marseilles remedy against the plague dating from 1722, Four Thieves Vinegar has continued to enjoy a reputation among her-balists as a mildly antiseptic but highly aromatic lotion. Supposedly once employed as a safeguard by four robbers who made a profes-sion of plundering the plague dead, it smells a little bit like rather exotic salad dressing as you will see if you try it.

Take ¼ ounce each of:

Calamus root	Ground nutmeg	Rue
Cinnamon	Lavender	Sage
Ground cloves	Mint	Wormwood
	Rosemary	

Place the herbs with 2 garlic heads, sliced, in a glass or ceramic container, and add 1 quart cider vinegar. Cover closely and keep at a warm temperature for 5 days. Strain, and add ¼ ounce powdered camphor before bottling for use.

Garlic Lotion

A simpler and really just as satisfactory traditional garlic lotion can be prepared thus: Infuse in 1 pint boiling white vinegar:

¼ ounce thyme	¼ ounce savory
¼ ounce sage	1 head garlic, sliced
¼ ounce hyssop	¼ cup salt
¼ ounce lavender	

Let this steep for at least 3 weeks before straining and bottling.

GOLDENROD
Solidago virgaurea

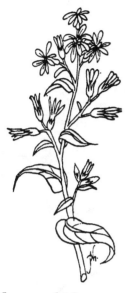

OTHER NAMES. *Solidago odora. Goldruthe.* Woundwort. Sweet-scented golden rod. Blue Mountain tea. Aaron's rod. *Verge d'or.*

HABITAT. Goldenrod grows throughout Central Asia, Europe, and North America, where, because of the delicious drink made from it, it is known as Blue Mountain tea. It is still a favorite ornamental "herbaceous border" plant in English country gardens. Although its leaves and tall (up to 5 feet) stems may die off in winter, its root is perennial. It bears alternating bright-green leaves, and the stems terminate in flat, bright golden-yellow masses of fragrant flowers which appear during the summer months. When bruised, both leaves and flowers give off a fragrance rather like wild carrot.

Goldenrod will do best in a dry soil in sun or partial sun.

PROPERTIES. Goldenrod contains tannin, and its aromatic and astringent qualities make it a gently stimulating digestive tea as well as a useful styptic lotion.

HOW TO USE IT.

Blue Mountain Tea

Infuse 1 teaspoon goldenrod leaves in a covered cup of boiling water. Strain and flavor with honey if desired.

HOPS
Humulus lupulus

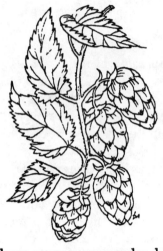

HABITAT. The hop plant was first mentioned by Pliny, who called it a garden plant and described how the Romans of his day ate it as we do the asparagus. It was not put to its chief use, however, the brewing of beer, until the fourteenth century. Before that time people drank mead or ale, beverages made out of fermented honey or barley and flavored with such herbs as ground ivy, marjoram, buck-bean, yarrow, germander, broom, or wormwood. Today the perennial hop grows wild in Europe, Britain, and western Asia, but is of course cultivated for beer in many temperate countries, including the United States. Herbalists generally buy their hop flowers from a supplier, but if you have a garden they are easy enough to grow for yourself. Being perennials, hops are nearly always grown from purchased roots rather than from seeds. These have to be obtained from companies who cater to vegetable growers and farmers, for the average nursery does not stock them.

Plant the hop root in a sunny spot thick end up in rich loamy soil in early spring, and stick one of those inexpensive cedar or redwood trellises obtainable from most nurseries in the ground behind it. Once the root begins to sprout, give it plenty of water, for the hop plant is a vine like the grape, and virtually cannot be overwatered. By midsummer you will have a luxurious tangle of square, downy stems covered with dark-green lobed leaves. In the axils of the leaves strongly aromatic flowers will appear, which contain the active property sought by the herbalist.

PROPERTIES. The female hop flower, a leafy yellow conelike catkin, contains the drug lupulin, which possesses tonic, diuretic, and sedative properties. Hop flowers have accordingly been employed by herbalists for various types of anodynes and sleeping potions for a very long time.

How TO USE IT.

Sedative Hop Tea

A mildly sedative hop infusion may be drunk before going to bed if you have trouble sleeping. Infuse 1 teaspoon dried hop flowers in 1 covered cup boiling water for 10 minutes. Strain and flavor with honey and lemon as required.

A Traditional Sleep Pillow

An old country remedy for restless slumbers is the hop pillow, a small pillow stuffed with hop flowers which have previously been sprinkled with a little alcohol to release their essential oil. Add a few rosebuds and verbena leaves for extra perfume if you like.

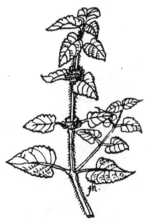

HOREHOUND, WHITE
Marrubium vulgare

OTHER NAMES. Marrubium. Hoarhound.

HABITAT. Horehound was known to the priests of the ancient Egyptians as seed of Horus, bull's blood, and eye of the star; it is also thought to have been marrob, one of the bitter herbs eaten by the Jews to commemorate the feast of Passover; the Romans gave it a high place in their herbal pharmacopoeia; Gerard recommends it as an antidote for "those that have drunk poyson or have been bitten of serpents."

Whatever its rumored value as an antidote, it is remarkably useful as an aid for coughs and colds.

Horehound grows wild all over Europe and the United States now, and is really very easy to cultivate. The usual method is by root division, but seeds or seedlings can be planted in spring. Plant in dryish soil, not overrich, and just make sure it gets a regular weeding. It possesses sectionally square, branching stems which may grow up to 1 foot or more, ending in white woolly-looking flowers in whorls, which will appear after the second year. The leaves are wrinkled, gray-green, and downy, and give off a curious musky odor when crushed.

PROPERTIES. Horehound contains, among other things, a bitter substance known as marrubium, essential oil, resin, tannin, and sugar. Its property as an expectorant makes it one of the favorite ingredients in herbal cough medicines. Combined with its bracing tonic effect, this property also makes it an excellent tonic tea for people suffering from colds.

HOW TO USE IT.

Horehound Tonic Tea

Infuse 1 teaspoon fresh or dried horehound leaves in 1 covered cup of boiling water. Strain and flavor with honey and a little ground ginger root if desired.

Horehound Tonic Blend

Take ½ ounce each of: Horehound
                        Rue
                        Hyssop
                        Licorice root
                        Marsh mallow root

Boil in 2 pints water until the quantity is reduced to 1½ pints. Strain and take in ½ teacup doses every 2 to 3 hours. (*Note:* Rue has been known to trigger mild allergic reactions in some people. I would advise those who know themselves to be liable to such symptoms to make use of the first simple horehound tea recipe given above.)

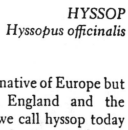

HYSSOP
Hyssopus officinalis

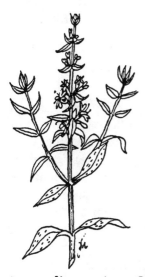

HABITAT. Originally a native of Europe but now naturalized in England and the United States, what we call hyssop today was probably not the herb eulogized by the Old Testament writer in the verse "Purge me with hyssop, and I shall be clean." *Hyssopus* means simply "a holy herb," and the plant referred to is now thought to have been marjoram.

However, today's hyssop also has fine aromatic qualities made use of both in perfumery and the manufacture of Chartreuse liquor (see Chapter 2), although the leaf will smell refreshingly bitter only if you try crushing it in your fingers. It is a very easy herb to grow, and will make an attractive, low (1 to 2 feet high) evergreen bush with whorls of red, blue, or white flowers if you keep it well trimmed. It does best in a warmish climate or sheltered position in full sun and a light, dry soil. If you plant it from seed or cutting, do it in spring; root division should be done in spring or fall.

PROPERTIES. Hyssop is used by herbalists for its powers as a stimulant, expectorant, aromatic, and diaphoretic and vermifuge (worm expeller). Many claim it has a special curative value for pulmonary diseases, and it is still used as a folk remedy for chronic rheumatism. The green herb, bruised and applied as a dressing, is found to heal bruises and cuts promptly.

HOW TO USE IT.

Hyssop Tea

Infuse 1 teaspoon dried hyssop leaves and flowers in 1 covered cup boiling water for 10 minutes. Strain and sweeten with honey. Drink up to 2 cups per day.

LAVENDER
Lavandula officinalis

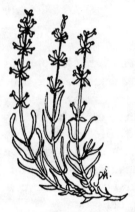

OTHER NAMES. English lavender. *Lavandula vera.*

HABITAT. Lavender is a hardy shrub originally indigenous to the Mediterranean area but now cultivated in gardens all over the world. In biblical times it was known as *nardos*, or nard, and Pliny recounts that the Romans payed as much as a hundred denarii [1] a pound for the blossoms. The Latin name *Lavandula* derives from the verb *lavare*, "to wash," for even in those times it was a favorite bath scent. From the time of the Tudors until today it has remained the primary ingredient in many soaps, perfumes, and colognes. The flowers are still used in country districts as a filling for sweet bags and sachets to place among the linens. Not only do they impart their fragrance, but they also serve as an excellent moth deterrent.

Lavender can be planted from seed in April, but the seeds take a long time to germinate. It is generally far easier to take cuttings or divide off roots from a parent plant. Root division should take place in spring, but cuttings can be taken at any time of the year. Make sure you take the cuttings from the newer shoots of the old bush. Plant them securely in well-drained, sandy soil in a sunny position, watering them well until they have begun to sprout. Once they develop into a small bush, prune the long flower stems back after flowering to ensure a strong, healthy growth the following year.

Lavender will grow as high as 3 feet if you let it, and its oblong grayish leaves and brush of pretty blue flower spikes can make a very fragrant and attractive garden hedge.

PROPERTIES. Lavender is rich in essential oils, notably linalool, cineol, pinene, limonene, geraniol, and borneol. It also contains a small amount of tannin. Herbalists of Gerard's day used lavender a lot as a condiment for flavoring dishes to comfort the stomach. It is now considered to possess aromatic and stimulating properties,

---

[1] About $10—over twice today's average price.

suitable for gently relieving fatigue when used externally in bath sachets or taken internally as an infusion.

How to use it.

Lavender Tea

A pleasant way to relieve nervous tension and exhaustion: Infuse 1 teaspoon dried, bruised lavender flowers in 1 covered cup boiling water for 15 minutes. Strain and flavor with honey if desired. Drink up to 1 cup per day.

LOVAGE
Levisticum officinale

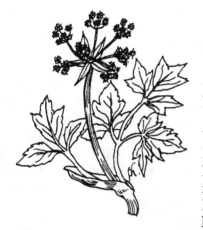

OTHER NAMES. *Ligusticum levisticum.* Lavose. Italian lovage. Old English lovage. Cornish lovage. Sea parsley.

HABITAT. Yet another herb brought westward by first the Romans, then the settlers of North America, lovage grows wild in the mountains of southern France, northern Greece, and the Balkans.

It is a good, hardy perennial, and grows with a thick, hollow stem like that of angelica, but more translucent and succulent. When crushed, the stem, leaves, and tiny yellow flowers give off an angelica-like perfume, while the delicious taste of the herb—for it is used in cooking—is halfway between that of parsley and celery.

When you grow your own lovage from seed, sow it in spring or fall in rich, moist soil in sun or partial sun. However, it is far quicker to propagate it by root division.

PROPERTIES. Lovage contains essential oils, angelic acid, a variety of resins, and a substance known as ligulin. An infusion is made from the herb whose action is aromatic, tonic, diuretic, and mildly stimulating. Some herbalists also consider it to be a useful emmenagogue, that is, an herb capable of bringing on the menstrual discharge in women.

How TO USE IT.

Lovage Tea

Infuse 1 ounce dried leaves, stems, and flowers in 1 pint boiling water. Cover closely. Strain after 15 minutes and flavor with honey if desired.

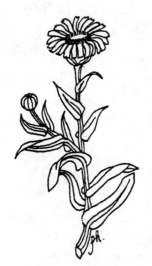

MARIGOLD
Calendula officinalis

OTHER NAMES. *Caltha officinalis*. Ruddes. Golds. Pot marigold. Marygold. Marybud. Holigold. Mary Gowles. *Oculus Christi. Solis sponsa*. Verrucaria. Jackanapes-on-horseback.

HABITAT. Possibly originating in India, the marigold is now a native of southern Europe, and a persistent self-seeding annual in gardens everywhere. The true calendula marigold, which should carefully be distinguished from the pungently scented tagetes, which is sold in many parts of the United States under the name marigold, possesses sectionally square stems with pale-green tongue-shaped leaves alternating upon them, and deep orange-gold flowers. It is extremely easy to grow from seed sown in late spring in a sunny or partially sunny position in your garden. Any type of soil will do. Flowers will appear by midsummer, and will probably continue to do so until the winter cold kills them off. Generally, they seed themselves without your even having to bother.

PROPERTIES. Marigold leaves and flowers, which should be gathered in the morning after the dew has dried off, contain phosphorus and vitamin C. In action they are astringent, stimulant, and perspiration-producing. Herbalists in the past used to use them to bring out measles and smallpox. Marigold flowers rubbed on wasp stings will help to alleviate the irritation, according to some country herbalists.

How to use it.
Marigold Infusion

As a lotion for bathing both cuts and abrasions, and as a stimulant tea, infuse 1 teaspoon dried flowers and leaves in 1 cup boiling water for 15 minutes. Strain and flavor with honey if desired. Drink up to 1 cup per day.

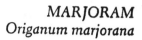

MARJORAM
Origanum marjorana

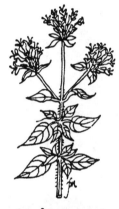

OTHER NAMES. Sweet marjoram. Knotted marjoram. *Marjorana hortensis.* Garden marjoram.

HABITAT. An ideal pot-herb, considered by the Romans sacred to beautiful Venus, goddess of love, marjoram is actually a native of Portugal. It is mentioned with great favor by Pliny, Gerard, Culpeper, and Parkinson, among others, as an excellent and useful plant, not only on account of its pharmaceutical and culinary values, but also for its strong and exquisite fragrance. It was used during the Middle Ages to strew the floors of hall and cottage alike, and turns up as an ingredient of many Elizabethan sweet bags. It also happens to make a fine herbal snuff.

Marjoram possesses a perennial root, although its leaves and stems frequently die off in winter in colder climates. The stems are transversely square, often purplish and downy, becoming woody at the base as the plant develops. The leaves are small, clear green, oval, and slightly downy on the undersides; the flowers appear as pale-lilac or grayish-white whorls or "knots." Dittany of Crete, an ornamental variety of marjoram, once used in flavoring and in sorcery (see Chapter 6), possesses grayer, more downy leaves, and pretty pink flowers.

If you wish to grow marjoram from seed, sow it in late spring in a reasonably moist soil in full sun. If you put it in the shade, its stems will grow long and straggly and grope pathetically toward the light!

Propagate by root division in the winter, and if you keep your plant in a pot take it indoors during frosty weather. Like the lavender, marjoram is quite amenable to being grown from stem cuttings also.

PROPERTIES. Marjoram contains an aromatic essential oil known by pharmacists as *oleum marjoranae*. Present-day herbalists consider the whole plant itself a stimulant and a tonic. An infusion of it known as spring tea is also thought to be excellent for any type of upset stomach.

HOW TO USE IT.

Spring Tea

Infuse 1 teaspoon dried leaves and tops of marjoram in 1 covered cup boiling water for 15 minutes. Strain and flavor with honey if desired. Up to 2 cups per day may be taken.

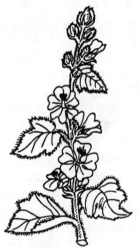

MARSH MALLOW
Althaea officinalis

OTHER NAMES. Sweet weed. Wymote. Mallards. Mauls. Schloss tea. Cheeses. Mortification root. Guimauve.

HABITAT. The marsh mallow and close botanical relatives, such as hollyhock, have been popular as table vegetables among the Egyptians, the Chinese, the Syrians, the Greeks, the Armenians, and the Romans for many centuries. Both Pliny and Dioscorides mention the marsh mallow in the context of medicinal herbs, however. Marsh mallow is native to Europe, southern England, western Asia, and North Africa and, as its name suggests, grows wild in damp ground, in ditches, beside rivers, and often near the sea. Although the marsh mallow can be raised from seed sown during the spring, propagation by cuttings or root division performed during the fall after the stalks have decayed is generally considered more satisfactory. Marsh mallow will take to any soil in any situation, provided it is kept reasonably moist. As the stems grow up to 4 feet tall, the plant should have at least 2 feet clearance on either side for adequate growth. The root is perennial, but the stems, the downy serrated leaves, and the large pink-purple flowers will die off each year. For medicinal purposes the leaves should be gathered singly as the flowers are coming into bloom.

PROPERTIES. Both the root and the leaves of the marsh mallow are used in herbal medicine. Both contain—but especially the root—a large quantity of mucilage (vegetable gum), some starch, a little pectin, asparagin, and sugar. On account of its mucilage, marsh mallow is used primarily as a demulcent and emollient (a substance for softening the skin and soothing external irritation). An infusion of the leaves is also used as cough medicine and a lotion for bathing sore eyes.

How TO USE IT.

Marsh-mallow Infusion

For soothing coughs, colds, and stomach upsets: Infuse 1 ounce dried leaves in 1 pint boiling water. Strain and flavor with honey if taken as a tea.

Marsh-mallow Compress

Steep the *fresh* leaves or fresh, bruised root of the marsh mallow in hot water and apply them to the affected part to reduce inflammation. Such a compress may also be used upon wasp stings.

MEADOWSWEET
Spiraea ulmaria

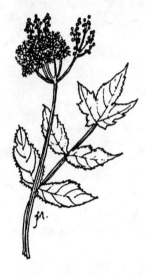

OTHER NAMES. *Filipendula ulmaria. Spiraea tomentosa.* Steeplebush. Meadsweet. Dollof. Queen of the meadow. Bridewort. Lady of the meadow.

HABITAT. Once held sacred by the Druids, meadowsweet became the favorite "strewing herb" of Queen Elizabeth I on account of its fragrance. "Queen Elizabeth of famous memory did more desire it than any other herb to strew her chambers withall," the seventeenth-century herbalist John Parkinson noted.

In its wild state, meadowsweet grows in damp fields and around streams. Its cream-colored, richly almond-scented tufts of flowers appear at the end of erect, purplish stems from which spring pairs of serrated, lobed leaves, dark green on top, pale and downy underneath. The lobes range in number from three to five. Although all parts of the herb carry its fragrance, it is concentrated chiefly in the flower, which from the sixteenth century onward was frequently used to scent wine and beer and provide the filling for linen sachets.

Meadowsweet is an easy herb to grow in your garden. It is as rewarding for its appearance as for its heady fragrance. The garden variety bears showy flowers of pink or deep rose and makes an attractive potted plant. Give it a moist, alkaline soil and a full or half day's sun.

PROPERTIES. Meadowsweet contains calcium, magnesium, iron, phosphorus, sodium, sulphur, and, most important, vitamin C. Herbalists find its action tonic, astringent, diuretic, and aromatic. It makes a delightfully scented diet drink which is also useful for aiding in recovery from feverish colds and digestive problems.

HOW TO USE IT.

Meadowsweet Tea

Infuse 1 teaspoon dried flowers, leaves, or root in 1 covered cup boiling water for 15 minutes. Strain and sweeten with honey. Drink 1 cup after meals.

MOTHERWORT
Leonurus cardiaca

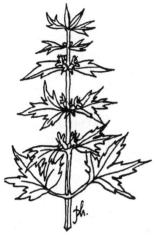

OTHER NAMES. Roman motherwort. Lion's tail. Throw-wort.

HABITAT. A native to many parts of Europe but now introduced to the United States, the motherwort, though primarily a garden plant, may be found growing wild in fields and under hedges. From a tough, perennial root it sends up square stems which may rise to a height of 3 feet. The leaves are close set and coarsely toothed and lobed, and the flowers, which appear during the summer months, are arranged in whorls of white, pink, or purple. When crushed, the leaves give off a pungent but aromatic odor. You may plant motherwort from seed or seedling in your garden, giving it full sun and about 12 inches on either side to grow. There are no special soil requirements; in fact, the plant will often seed itself if allowed to.

PROPERTIES. Old herbalists used to claim that there was no better herb for strengthening and gladdening the heart, as the Latin name, *Leonurus cardiaca*, would indeed suggest. Motherwort possesses value as a perspiration producer, a tonic, a stimulant, and, according to many herbalists, an emmenagogue. It is said to allay nervous irritability and provide stimulus without any of the "shakes" which often accompany such drugs as caffeine.

HOW TO USE IT.

Motherwort Tonic Infusion

Motherwort possesses a pungent and, to some, unpleasant taste. It is therefore advisable to mix a small amount of aromatic herb or spice similar in effect to motherwort's with your infusion—lavender, for example.

Infuse 1 teaspoon dried tops and leaves of motherwort in 1 cup boiling water for 15 minutes. Strain and flavor with honey if desired. Take up to 1 cup per day.

MULLEIN
Verbascum thapsus

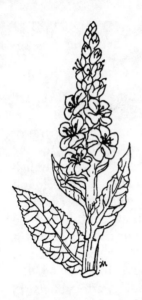

OTHER NAMES. Torches. Velvet dock. Velvet plant. Flannel leaf. Woolen. Rag paper. Candlewick plant. Wild ice leaf. Clown's lungwort. Aaron's rod. Jupiter's staff. Jacob's staff. Peter's staff. Shepherd's staff. Clot. Duffle. Feltwort. Hag's taper.

HABITAT. An age-old reputed banisher of demons and a sharer of garlic's reputation as the plant that guarded Ulysses from Circe's witchery, mullein is found growing in the Himalayas, on the eastern seaboard of the United States, and throughout Europe and the British Isles.

As some of its other names suggest, it grows tall and straight, frequently to a majestic 5 feet. Its broad, woolly leaves and flat pale-yellow or white flowers are set closely about the thick stem. The garden variety of mullein, however (*phoenicum*), produces purple blossoms. Mullein, a hardy biennial, will grow in practically any soil with reasonably little attention and general watering. It does best, however, in full sun. It will often seed itself if left to its own devices. The leaves and the flowers, the parts used in herbal medicine, possess the most potency when gathered during the summer months.

PROPERTIES. Mullein contains mucilage, resin, tannin, an essential oil, and a variety of mineral salts, notably those of potassium, iron, magnesium, and sulphur. Its chief uses are as a sedative, demulcent and emollient, and astringent, although country herbalists still make poultices for toothache and neuralgia from it. The decoction is not only handy to soothe coughs and prevent expectoration, but is also said to relieve the pain and irritation of hemorrhoids.

HOW TO USE IT.
Mullein Decoction
Boil 1 ounce dried mullein leaves in 1 pint milk in a covered

container for 10 minutes. Strain and flavor with honey if desired. Take 1 wineglass 3 times daily.
Mullein Tea

A mildly sedative, plain infusion of mullein leaves may also be used to almost the same effect:

Infuse 1 teaspoon dried leaves in 1 cup boiling water. Take up to 2 cups per day.

Note: As mullein leaves have, to some, a rather pungent odor, it is frequent practice to include an aromatic spice such as cloves or cinnamon in recipes where it is to be taken internally.
Mullein Inhalation

To help clear the sinus passages after a cold, try infusing ½ ounce mullein herb in a kettle of boiling water and inhaling the steam. You may also add a few sticky poplar buds, known in the United States as balm of Gilead, for extra aromatic effect.

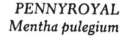

PENNYROYAL
Mentha pulegium

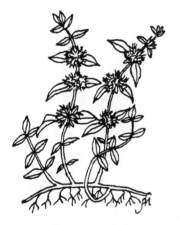

OTHER NAMES. *Hedeoma pulegioides.* Tickweed. Squawmint (U.S.). Run-by-the-ground. Lurk-in-the-ditch. Pudding grass. Piliolerial.

HABITAT. The Greeks used to give pennyroyal potions to prospective candidates for initiation into the mysteries of Eleusis; they considered it to be sacred to Demeter, the goddess of nature, in whose honor the mysteries were celebrated. It is the smallest of all the mints, and was the first to be cultivated. Pliny, Dioscorides, the Cymry of Wales, the Anglo-Saxon leeches, and even the medieval monks all treasured this little herb for its botanical virtues. Not only do its leaves contain a powerful stimulant, but they and the essential oil derived from them are extremely effective for keeping fleas and mosquitoes away. They are, in fact, an old camper's standby. Like most other mints save catnip, pennyroyal does best in damp ground, and is very easily grown from cuttings or by root division. Again like most other mints, it requires strict control, or its runners will start popping up in all kinds of unexpected, and probably unwanted, places. If you allow it to, it will form a very attractive carpet, for the leaves tend to get smaller as the plant gets larger. The faintly downy leaves themselves grow on short stalks on either side of the main transversely square stem. They are more oval than oblong in-shape and of a grayish-green color. The flower clusters appear in typical mintlike whorls and range in color from purple to pale lilac.

PROPERTIES. Pennyroyal contains oil of pulegium, a powerfully aromatic essential oil from which its virtues are derived. Herbalists use it as a diaphoretic, an aromatic, an emmenagogue, and a stimulant. It is also beneficial for nausea, flatulence, and stomach upsets.

HOW TO USE IT.

Pennyroyal Tea

Infuse 1 teaspoon dried pennyroyal tops and leaves in 1 covered cup boiling water. Strain and flavor with honey if required. Take warm as frequently as desired.

PEPPERMINT
Mentha piperita

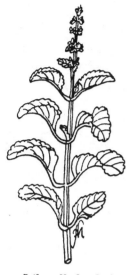

OTHER NAMES. Brandy mint. Lammint.

HABITAT. A native of Europe and the United States, peppermint crowned the heads of both the Greeks and the Romans when they feasted, adorned their tables, and flavored their wines and sauces—or so Pliny said. There also exists evidence that it was cultivated by the ancient Egyptians. But although peppermint appears in Icelandic herbals of the thirteenth century, it seems to have come into general use in Western Europe only during the eighteenth, and was introduced first in England.

Like all the Labiatae mint family, peppermint will grow best in moist soil, in sun or shade. Its transversely square stem can grow as high as 3 feet. Its leaves are lance-shaped, smooth, toothed, and dark green, sometimes almost purple in color, with downy veins on the undersides. The whorled flowers are small and range from pale violet to purple in color. Plant from root or underground runner for quickest results, and again beware: you have a very willful and persistent herb on your hands.

PROPERTIES. Peppermint contains probably the most important essential oil in the entire herbal pharmocopoeia: menthol. It also contains traces of a variety of others, among which are numbered pinene, cineol, and limonene. The herb acts primarily as an aromatic and a stimulant. Peppermint tea is an excellent aid toward remedying an upset stomach, frayed nerves, and an incipient cold.

HOW TO USE IT.

Peppermint Tea (Stimulant)

Infuse 1 teaspoon dried leaves and tops in 1 covered cup boiling water for 10 minutes. Strain and flavor with honey if required. Take as often as needed.

Traditional Peppermint Cold Cure

To be taken at the onset of a cold.

Mix equal quantities of dried peppermint, elder flowers, and yarrow. Infuse 1 teaspoon in 1 covered cup boiling water for 15 minutes. Strain, flavor with honey, and drink hot.

Peppermint Sedative I

    Mix equal parts of: Peppermint
                              Wood betony (*Betonica officinalis*)
                              Caraway seed

Infuse 1 teaspoonful in 1 covered cup boiling water for 15 minutes; strain and sweeten with honey if desired. Take up to 1 cup before going to bed.

Peppermint Sedative II

    Another aid against insomnia also using betony is the following old recipe:

    Mix equal parts of: 1 ounce finely cut dried peppermint herb
                              ½ ounce rue herb
                              ½ ounce wood betony (*Betonica officinalis*)

Infuse 1 teaspoon in 1 covered cup boiling water for 15 minutes; strain and sweeten, and drink before going to bed. However, before using this recipe please read the section dealing with rue.

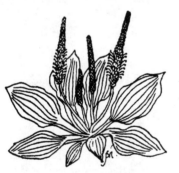

PLANTAIN
Plantago major

OTHER NAMES. *Plantago lanceolate.* Ripple grass. Waybread. Waybroad. Slan-lus. Snake-weed. Cuckoo's bread. Englishman's foot. Soldier's herb.

HABITAT. Well, we can all see why people in Australia and New Zealand call it Englishman's foot. (Actually, the legend really says that wherever the English have set foot plantain is sure to rise.) Although an unattractive herb and as much of a lawn nuisance to the gardener as the dandelion, plantain has enjoyed a reputation among old herbalists as a cure-all for poisons and snakebite since the time of the Saxons. "And thou Weybroed [plantain], Mother of Herbs, open from the East, mighty within ..." runs one of the incantations from the Nine Herbs Charm, calling on the herb to lend its power to the healer. "If a wood hound [mad dog] rend a man," says a later herbal jauntily, "take this wort [herb], rub it fine and lay it on; then will the spot soon be whole!"

Plantain is a ubiquitous herb, native to northern and Central Asia, Europe, the British Isles, and the United States. It grows just about anywhere: field, roadside, or garden. Its rosette of broad longitudinally veined leaves with channeled stems radiating from a single center is practically unmistakable. Tiny off-white blossoms tinged with green and purple cluster about the erect flower spikes during the summer.

PROPERTIES. Plantain seeds are rich in mucilage, and have been quite effectively employed as a substitute for linseed to make oil. They are also one of the primary ingredients of birdseed. The plant itself contains sulphur, calcium and potassium, and its astringent qualities have made it valuable as a vulnerary for all these centuries.

HOW TO USE IT.

Plaintain Infusion

An old herbal remedy for diarrhea:

Infuse 1 ounce dried plantain leaves in 1 part boiling water. Cover and let stand in a warm place for 20 minutes, then strain and let cool. Take 1 wineglass to ½ teacup 3 or 4 times daily.

Plantain Compress

For the relief of minor cuts, swellings, scratches, and abrasions:

Bruise fresh, clean plantain leaves well, and apply to the affected area.

PRIMROSE
Primula veris

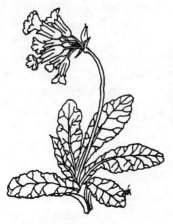

OTHER NAMES. Cowslip. Butter rose. Herb peter. Paigle. Peggle. Key flower. Keys of heaven. Fairy cups. Petty mulleins. Crewel. Buckles. Palsywort. Plumrocks. Mayflower. Password. Artetyke. Drelip. Our Lady's keys. Arthritica. *Cuy lippe.*

HABITAT. A native of the British Isles and once sacred to Freya, the northern love goddess, the primrose was hastily passed into the possession of Our Lady with the advent of Christianity. In either case, however, it was still the "keys of heaven." Its Latin name indicates, quite truly, that it is also "the first little flower of spring," a familiar sight in many gardens in Europe and the United States. Its "keys" are its pendant bell-shaped flowers of yellow or shades of red and purple in garden varieties.

Primroses are perennial, and bear long oval wrinkled leaves of a bright-green color which spring from a common base; the flowers themselves are borne upon a separate stem which rises among and usually above the leaves. You can best grow primroses from root division done in the fall. If you wish to raise them from seed, use a moist, light potting mix, plenty of watering and half sun or shade.

PROPERTIES. Primrose contains a fragrant essential oil and two active principles known as primulin and saponin. Its action is antispasmodic, astringent, and in strong doses vermifuge and emetic.

HOW TO USE IT.

Primrose Tea

"Primrose tea," says Gerard, "drunk in the month of May is famous for curing the phrensie"! It is still used by herbalists as a fragrant sedative for banishing headaches:

Infuse 1 teaspoon dried, chopped primrose leaves and flowers in 1 cup boiling water. Cover closely and let stand for 10 minutes. Strain and sweeten with honey if required. Drink up to 1 cup per day.

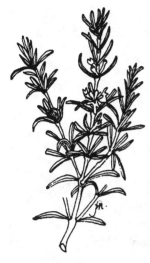

ROSEMARY
Rosmarinus officinalis

OTHER NAMES. Incensier. *Rosmarinus coronarium.*

HABITAT. An old favorite of the Greeks, brought west by the Romans, and used during the Middle Ages as an incense when frankincense was rare, rosemary has been celebrated in myth, magic, and herbal medicine for many centuries. When Shakespeare has Ophelia say, "There's rosemary, that's for remembrance," she is simply giving voice to an age-old belief that rosemary actually strengthened the memory, whether taken internally or hung from the rafters. It was accordingly incorporated in wreaths and posies both at weddings and at funerals, and presented in festive bouquets on New Year's Day, "lest old acquaintance be forgot."

Rosemary is an evergreen perennial, and will grow into a shrub or hedge depending on how you trim it. The easiest way to grow it is by root division in the fall or 6-inch cuttings taken in August and planted with half to two thirds of their length in the ground. Ideally it should have a dry, sandy soil, a sheltered position, and plenty of sun.

PROPERTIES. Rosemary is rich in tannic acid, camphorous resin, and an essential oil containing borneol and bornyl acetate. It is used as an aromatic, a tonic, an astringent, and a stimulant. Rosemary infusions are an old herbal standby for relieving tension headaches; they also happen to make one of the best hair rinses known! (See Chapter 3.)

HOW TO USE IT.

Rosemary Tea (Stimulant and Antidepressive)

Infuse 1 teaspoon dried rosemary tops, leaves, or flowers in 1 covered cup boiling water for 10 minutes. Strain and flavor with honey to taste. Drink while still warm as often as required.

Similar in effect and equally fragrant is:

Rosemary Wine

Steep a handful of chopped fresh sprigs of rosemary direct from the garden in a bottle of white wine for 3 days. Strain and decant for use. Try it. It's delicious.

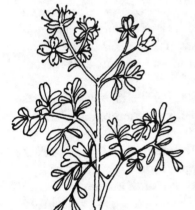

RUE
Ruta graveolens

OTHER NAMES. Herb of grace. Garden rue. German rue.

HABITAT. A powerful old favorite of the witches of Florence, rue has been for many centuries included on the same list of "demonofuges" as such plants as angelica, dill, and garlic. Because of its dual action as disinfectant and flea repellent—insects are said to stay far from it—rue was once strewn about the floors of law courts in an attempt to prevent the spread of jail fever, frequently carried to the bar by prisoners fresh from the appallingly squalid jails of the day.

Rue is a native of Italy and southern Europe, but is grown in herb gardens throughout Europe and the United States. It is a hardy evergreen perennial, and its woody stem can grow as high as 3 feet. Its interesting gray-green, much divided leaves and bright-yellow flowers will make an intriguing addition to your herb garden, and it is really a remarkably easy and undemanding plant to grow. In fact, in rue's case, the poorer the soil, the better the plant! Seed or plant cuttings in spring, in damp, shady soil to begin with until the seedlings have really taken hold. Then transfer them to an open patch of ground with plenty of sun. Remember, it is a southern plant, and an herb's original habitat can tell you a lot about the conditions it will do best in.

PROPERTIES. Rue is rich in a considerably powerful stimulant vegetable drug known as rutin. Herbalists use rue as a stimulant, an antispasmodic (an herb which helps to prevent muscular spasms and contractions), and an emmenagogue. Because of its powerful action, rue should always be used *cautiously*, and never taken to excess. In some instances the herb has been known to produce an allergic rash on the skin of the handler.

How to use it.

Rue Tea

A bitter though aromatic and stimulating drink not to be taken in excess of 1 cup per day:

Infuse 1 teaspoon fresh herbs (dried is less powerful) in 1 covered cup boiling water for 5 minutes. Strain and flavor with honey to taste. Drink *cold* between meals as a stimulant. Drink *hot* as an emmenagogue. Do not take immediately after meals, as rue has been known to have an emetic effect.

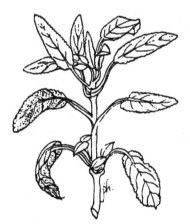

SAGE
Salvia officinalis

Other names. Sawge. Garden sage. *Salvia salvatrix.*

Habitat. Sage is a tough evergreen perennial originating from the northern Mediterranean shores. Its name derives from the Latin *salvere*, to save or be well, and it has long been thought to have possessed remarkable life-prolonging virtues. "*Cur moriatur homo cui salvia crescit in horto?*" (Why should a man die who has sage growing in his garden?), says one old proverb. Like so many herbs, sage was taken over from the Greek physicians by the Romans, who brought it west with them in their travels of conquest, although a general knowledge of its uses only arrived later with the various editions of Apuleius and Dioscorides.

Sage comes in many varieties, all equally useful to the herbalist. Garden sage, the most commonly grown one, possesses gray-green finely wrinkled leaves, slightly downy and rounded at the tips. They grow in pairs upon the stem and give out a strong aromatic fragrance shared by the spikes of blue or purple flowers when you crush them in your fingers. Bees love it! Plant seeds or cuttings in the spring in dryish soil with plenty of sun; the really dedicated gardener will bank them with manure and mulch during the winter, but this is really not necessary in warmer climates. Just a little fertilizer from time to time is all your herbs will ever need.

PROPERTIES. Garden sage is rich in a hydrocarbon all its own known as salvene. Also present in lesser amounts are those other common essential-oil components borneol, pinene, cineol, and thujone. The last is a potent preservative which strongly resists bacterial decomposition in animal tissues. In action, sage is astringent, aromatic, stimulant, and bitterly tonic. It is employed extensively in gargles, mouthwashes, vulneraries, febrifuges, poultices, smoking mixtures, tooth powders, hair dyes, blood purifiers, and emmenagogues, not to mention cooking.

How TO USE IT.

Simple Infusion

As a mouthwash to aid bleeding gums or a tea to help relieve nervous headaches, infuse 1 teaspoon dried leaves and tops of sage in 1 covered cup boiling water (1 ounce to 1 pint if a greater quantity is needed). Strain after 10 minutes and sweeten with honey if you are drinking it as a tea.

Astringent Mouthwash

For a more astringent mouthwash, place 2 ounces dried leaves and tops of sage in a covered enamel or Pyrex container and infuse it in 1 pint boiling malt vinegar for 30 minutes. Strain and dilute with 1 pint water before use.

Gargle

To compose a gargle with sage, decoct (simmer) for 5 minutes 6 sage leaves placed in a nonmetallic pot in 1 dessertspoon clover honey, 1 tablespoon light vinegar, and 1 small glass port wine.

Febrifuge

An ideal aromatic drink to help bring down the temperature of those laid up in bed with colds or flu is the following:

Infuse half an ounce of dried sage tops and leaves in 1 quart boiling water. Add the juice of 1 lemon and 1 ounce sugar or honey. Stir well; cover tightly for 30 minutes. Strain and take as often as required, warm or cold.

1857 Sage Poultice

Again making use of sage's excellent aromatic, astringent, and antibacterial properties is the following nineteenth-century poultice recipe for soothing sprains:

Bruise a handful of fresh sage leaves and boil them in a gill (¼ pint) of vinegar for 5 minutes; apply this in a folded napkin as hot as can be borne to the part affected.

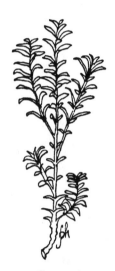

SAVORY
Satureia hortensis

OTHER NAMES. Bean herb. *Bohnenkraut.*

HABITAT. Summer savory and its close relative, winter savory *(Satureia montana),* belong to the plant family Satureiae, comprising around fourteen different aromatic herbs. The Roman poet Virgil wrote glowingly of both winter and summer savory and recommended their use as a bee herb to plant around the hives. Not only does the fragrance attract the bees, but the juice of the leaf brings quick relief when rubbed on bee stings. The Latin name *Satureia* was first used by Pliny, and seems to indicate some connection—possibly their beekeeping propensities—between the herb and satyrs, horned and hoofed phallic demigods once thought to inhabit the ancient Greek countryside. Of the two varieties, summer and winter savory, summer is thought to be the most powerful for herbal medicine. It should be ideally planted in light but rich soil in full sun. Whereas summer savory is only an annual, winter savory is perennial and will go on growing happily throughout the year. Just make sure to keep the stems clipped to prevent them from growing woody and straggly during the winter months. As the seeds of both varieties take rather long to germinate, it is advisable to plant from seedlings, or propagate from a parent plant by root division or cuttings. Plant savory toward the front of your herb garden, for it rarely grows taller than 12 inches high. Both savories are easily recognizable, having short, oblong leaves spring-ing directly from their stems which give off a musky fragrance when crushed, and bearing pale lilac flowers during the summer months.

PROPERTIES. Savory, though used chiefly as a cooking herb, also possesses aromatic and digestive properties. Culpeper recom-mended it for "colic," and it is still used as a digestive tea to this day.

HOW TO USE IT.

Savory Tea

To ease cramps caused by indigestion, infuse 1 teaspoon dried savory leaves in 1 covered cup boiling water for 10 minutes. Strain and sweeten with honey, as required. Take 1 cup warm or lukewarm as often as needed.

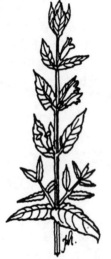

SKULLCAP
Scutellaria galericulata (European variety)
Scutellaria lateriflora (American variety)

OTHER NAMES. Greater skullcap. Mad-dog skullcap. Madweed. Helmet flower. Hood-wort. Toque.

HABITAT. Ubiquitous and particularly prevalent in the United States, this distant relative of the mints is highly valued as one of the finest sedatives in the pharmacopoeia. Its old American names mad-dog skullcap and madweed are indicative of the uses it has been put to in the past as a remedy for hydrophobia, convulsions, and St. Vitus's dance.

In its wild state, skullcap seems to favor damp, shady situations beside streams or ponds, but in cultivation will take to half shade and a regular soil. Propagation by root division or seed should be done in March or April, and the herb should be given 6 inches on either side of it in which to spread out.

The stem of the skullcap is sectionally square like all Labiatae, its root perennial, and its leaves oblong and tapering, slightly downy and notched. The flowers grow in pairs from the leaf axils and are blue and vaguely helmet-shaped; hence the English names hoodwort and helmet flower, and the French one, toque.

PROPERTIES. Tannin, cellulose, but more especially the essential oil scutellarin make skullcap one of the most useful natural nervines yet discovered. It has been given for hysteria, convulsions, rickets, St. Vitus' dance, hydrophobia, and neuralgia. It makes a highly efficacious sedative tea.

HOW TO USE IT.

Skullcap Infusion

For a tonic and calming tea, infuse 1 teaspoon dried and powdered herb in 1 covered cup of boiling water for 10 minutes. Strain and sweeten with honey as required. Drink up to 2 cups per day in ½-cup doses.

A Traditional Skullcap Blend

For relief from nervous headaches, mix:

> 1 part dried skullcap
> 1 part peppermint
> 1 part sage

Infuse 1 teaspoonful in 1 covered cup boiling water for 10 minutes. Strain and sweeten to taste. Drink 1 warm cup as often as needed.

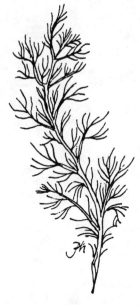

SOUTHERNWOOD
Artemisia abrotanum

OTHER NAMES. Lad's love. Old man. Boy's love. Appleringie. *Garde-robe.* Maiden's ruin.

HABITAT. The names boy's love and maiden's ruin tell a story all by themselves. Indeed the sexual stimulants said to be resident in southernwood made it a frequent ingredient for supposedly beard-producing ointments and not so innocent posies of wildflowers bestowed by country lads upon their lasses. Be that as it may. Southernwood was a favorite old monastic herbary plant which was brought to England from its native Mediterranean habitat in 1548. As it is an evergreen perennial, it is used fairly extensively in English flower gardens as a border plant. Its finely divided gray-green leaves give off a delicious tangy, lemony smell when crushed, which incidentally is highly offensive to bees and moths. On this account it makes a useful and time-honored filling for linen-sachets, hence *garde-robe,* the French name for the herb.

Southernwood will grow as tall as 5 feet if you let it and is best grown from root division accomplished in the spring or fall. It does best in a light, sandy soil with full sun.

PROPERTIES. Like its cousin wormwood, southernwood is rich in a substance known to pharmacists as absinthol, the primary ingredient of the French drink absinthe. Southernwood is used chiefly as an emmenagogue and on this account it is interesting to speculate whether the herb's names lad's love and maiden's ruin pertain more to a more specific and known use than merely to a quaint rustic ritual, although it also possesses stimulating tonic, vermifuge, and antiseptic properties.

HOW TO USE IT.
Southernwood Tea
To make a strong stimulant tea, infuse 1 ounce dried southern-

wood leaves and tops in 1 pint boiling water. Cover closely for 10 minutes, then strain and flavor with honey to taste. Use with caution.

SPEARMINT
Mentha viridis

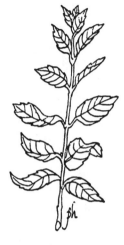

OTHER NAMES. Garden mint. Mackerel mint. Our Lady's mint. Green mint. Spire mint. Sage of Bethlehem. *Erba Santa Maria. Menthe de Notre Dame. Frauen munze.*

HABITAT. Theophrastus of Eresus tells us that the word *mentha* is really the name of an unlucky nymph who fell afoul of Persephone, the Greek goddess of the dead, on account of the interest Hades, Persephone's husband, showed in her. She was quickly transformed into a plant—spearmint to be exact—by the jealous goddess, which Hades perversely continued to hold particularly dear from that time onward.

Spearmint's sinister underworld connections notwithstanding, it became a treasured perfume in Greek and Roman times, frequently being used to scent bath water. The Romans brought it westward with them, and the first settlers took it with them to America, where it now runs wild. Both Gerard and Parkinson extolled mint's virtues highly, and Culpeper mentions almost forty separate ailments ranging from sore throat to dandruff, for which he considered spearmint to be "singularly good."

Spearmint grows with sectionally square, erect stems typical of the Labiatae family. The leaves are green, shiny, fine-toothed, and lance-shaped, and beneath them the veins are sharply delineated. When crushed they yield the strong, characteristic odor of spearmint. The flowers are tiny whorls of pink or lilac clustering about a tapering spike. A hardy perennial, spearmint flourishes best in moist soil, in partial sun or shade. It is most easily grown from root runners taken from another plant.

PROPERTIES. Spearmint contains a strongly aromatic essential oil much used in perfumery and cookery. The most important natural chemical components of this oil are carvone and limonene. Spearmint's chief uses for the herbalist are as a stimulant, an antispasmodic, and a digestive. It is also extremely useful for combating nausea and vomiting, and makes a fragrant tea helpful to sufferers from colds or flu, but delicious on any occasion.

HOW TO USE IT.

Simple Spearmint Tea

Infuse 1 teaspoon dried spearmint leaves and tops in one covered cup of boiling water for ten minutes. Strain and flavor with honey to taste. Drink warm or cold, as often as required.

Two Digestive Spearmint Tea Blends

1. Mix equal amounts spearmint, fennel, dill, anise, camomile, and catnip. Infuse 1 teaspoon in 1 covered cup boiling water for 15 minutes. Strain and drink slowly, flavored with honey if required.

2. Mix equal amounts spearmint, catnip, camomile, and valerian. Infuse 1 teaspoon in 1 covered cup boiling water for 15 minutes. Strain, flavor with honey, and drink warm every 2 hours.

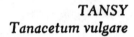

TANSY
Tanacetum vulgare

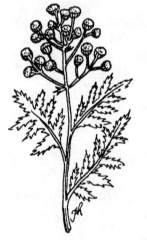

OTHER NAMES. Buttons. Bitter buttons. Parsley fern.

HABITAT. Tansy was the herb given to Jupiter's cupbearer Ganymede to make him immortal. In fact the Greek word *athanaton*, from which *Tanacetum* derives, means "deathless." Whether this name may be traced to Ganymede's story or simply to the fact that tansy was an herb once used by the ancients for embalming is a matter of opinion, although I suspect the latter.

Tansy grows wild all over Europe and the United States. It is a hardy perennial which takes to a chalky soil, and can often be found at roadsides and in waste ground. It grows to a height of 2 to 3 feet, and its much-divided leaves grow alternately upon the stem. Its flowers are buttonlike and bright yellow, and all parts of it yield an aromatic lemon fragrance when crushed.

You can grow tansy from seed or by root division in any soil, but it does need full sun. Although the leaves die off in winter, the root will send up new shoots the following year.

PROPERTIES. Tansy is a potent herb and should be used with caution. It contains tannin, resin, an essential oil composed mainly of thujone (one of the chemical components of sage), and a substance peculiar to the plant, tanacetin. It is used in herbalism as a tonic, a vermifuge, a diaphoretic, a stimulant, a poultice for sprains, and, most important, an emmenagogue. In moderate doses the herb exercises a benign and tonic effect, but in larger ones a violently irritating and narcotic one. So let me repeat: use it with caution.

HOW TO USE IT.

Tansy Tea

Infuse 1 ounce dried tansy leaves and tops in 1 pint boiling water. Cover closely for 10 minutes before straining. Flavor with honey to taste, and take in small wineglass doses.

THYME
Thymus vulgaris

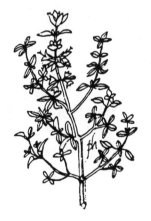

OTHER NAMES. Common thyme. Garden thyme.

HABITAT. Thyme is a shrubby herb which grows wild all over the low hills of the Mediterranean regions, Asia Minor, and Greece. It was introduced to England sometime before the sixteenth century. It possesses a woody perennial root from which spring many thin-branching stems which grow hard and twiglike with age. The paired leaves are tiny, oval, and gray-green in color, and the flowers grow in pale-purple whorls. Both give off a spicy, incenselike perfume highly attractive to bees, and indeed the word "thyme" itself derives from the Greek meaning "to fumigate."

There are any number of varieties of thyme, all possessing similar herbal properties: broad-leafed thyme, narrow-leafed thyme, French thyme, woolly thyme, creeping thyme—the list goes on forever. They all require a light, well-drained soil and full sun if possible. Cuttings or seeds may be planted in late spring or early summer; the bush should be kept in trim regularly with a pair of sheers or scissors to ensure healthy growth. Fork the surrounding earth well in the fall and bank new soil around the roots, making sure they are free of weeds.

PROPERTIES. Thyme contains two invaluable chemical substances, thymol and carvacrol. Like thujone in sage, thymol is a powerful preservative and antibacterial agent, although herbalists use thyme as not only an antiseptic but a tonic, an aromatic digestive, and a diaphoretic as well. Thyme sachets are said to be effective in keeping the moths away from linen closets.

How TO USE IT.

Thyme Tea

For headache, sore throat, coughs, and indigestion, infuse 1 teaspoon dried leaves and tops of thyme (to which a pinch of rosemary may be added), in 1 covered cup boiling water for 10 minutes. Strain and flavor with honey. Drink as often as required.

Thyme Poultice

Mix together:

> 2 ounces camomile
> 2 ounces lavender
> 1 ounce thyme
> 1 large pinch ground cloves

Enclose 2½ ounces of the herb mixture in a sachet and soak it in hot water for 2 minutes. Apply it to the bruised or swollen part as hot as possible without scalding.

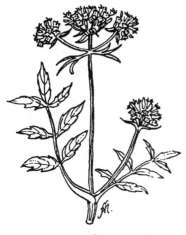

VALERIAN
Valeriana officinalis

OTHER NAMES. All-heal. Phu. Amantilla. Setwall. Setewale. Capon's tail. St. George's herb. Garden heliotrope. Fragrant valerian. Vandal root. Great wild valerian.

HABITAT. Valerian is a tall, straight perennial with a round hollow grooved stem that emerges from a short tuberous root set in a tangle of lesser rootlets. Its light-green serrated, paired leaves tend to stay close to the ground, and it produces small and fragrant pink, blue, or white flowers which gather in bunches at the end of the stalks.

However, its one unpleasant quality is the rest of the plant's smell. Both Galen and Dioscorides gave valerian the name "phu," and it is indeed well given, for the odor of the leaves, stems, and particularly the root is extremely pungent and unpleasant. Cats and rats, however, delight in it. On this account, some herbalists have suggested that valerian was the secret of the legendary Pied Piper of Hamlin's irresistible power over rats! If he did indeed possess a secret, however, it was far more likely to have been oil of rhodium, a time-honored extract from a type of convolvulus plant which exerts an extraordinary attractive power over rats.

To propagate valerian, use seeds or root division; it puts out underground runners, and these may be easily snipped off and replanted in a suitable spot. Valerian is not a demanding herb. It requires no special soil, only regular watering, and as much sun as you can provide.

PROPERTIES. Valerian's impressive properties are all vested in its root, which contains valerianic acid and two vegetable drugs known to herbal pharmacists as chatarine and valerianine. Valerian root is a powerful nerve stimulant and antispasmodic. Paradoxically, its greatest and most effective use among herbalists is as a sedative and pain-killer. The purified extract is also employed as a specific for epilepsy.

HOW TO USE IT.

Valerian tea is a time-honored herbal antidote for insomnia. In ordinary doses it exerts an extraordinary pacifying influence ("Men who begin to fight and when you wish to stop them, give to them the juice of *amantilla id est valerian* and peace will be made immediately," says one fifteenth-century herbal). However, in large or too-frequent doses valerian is dangerous, producing exactly the reverse effects required: headache, vertigo, nervous agitation, muscular spasms, and even hallucinations. It should accordingly be used with caution and discretion.

Valerian Tea

Infuse 1 teaspoon powdered valerian root in 1 pint boiling water for 10 minutes in a covered glass or ceramic pot. Strain and flavor with an aromatic spice such as mace, and add honey to taste. Take up to 1 cup a day before retiring.

VERBENA
Lippia citriodora

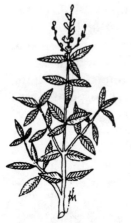

OTHER NAMES. *Aloysia citriodora.* Lemon verbena. Lemon-scented verbena. Verveine citronella. *Verveine odorante. Verbena triphylla. Lippia triphylla.* Herb Louisa.

HABITAT. Verbena's native habitat is Peru and Chile, but it was introduced to England and North America by the Spanish during the eighteenth century—relatively recently for an herb. It is a perennial but deciduous shrub which may grow to a height of 6 feet under ideal conditions if allowed. It bears narrow leaves generally in sets of three on a light-colored woody stem, and its tiny white or pale lilac flowers grow on spikes. Its herbal value lies in its leaves, which if even lightly brushed against—let alone crushed—give off an almost overpowering scent of lemons.

Verbena has good credentials as a candidate for your herb garden, especially if you are a lazy gardener like me. Just plant it in regular, well-drained soil with as much sun as you can. If you have a sunny wall in your garden, plant it against that. It can be raised from seed or seedling, or better still from cuttings. Clip back the straggly parts in spring if you wish to keep your verbena looking bushy.

PROPERTIES. Verbena owes its properties to its essential oils, which make it useful as a digestive like balm and the mints. However, whereas peppermint and spearmint used by themselves are stimulants, verbena is a mild sedative and cooling febrifuge. It can be taken in the form of either a decoction or a fragrant and delicious infusion.

HOW TO USE IT.

Verbena Tea

Infuse 1 teaspoon dried verbena leaves and tops in 1 covered cup boiling water for 15 minutes. Strain and flavor with honey to taste. Drink after meals as often as required.

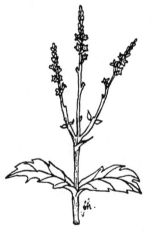

VERVAIN
Verbena officinalis

OTHER NAMES. Herb of grace. *Herba veneris. Herbe sacrée.*

HABITAT. Once used by the Druids and Romans for sprinkling holy water, vervain was inherited by later sorcerers and wise women, who made frequent use of it in their magical rituals. The Elizabethans mixed it in love philters and cosmetics, and Florentine witches used it as a good-luck charm. Herbalists use it today as a febrifuge, tonic, and expectorant. In the United States its close relative *Verbena hastata*, otherwise known as blue vervain, wild or Indian hyssop, and simpler's joy, is used to similar effect.

Vervain grows wild in meadows and hedgerows throughout Europe, the United States, and the Far East. It is a perennial herb, with a sectionally square stem, pale-green, odorless, serrated leaves growing opposite one another, and spikes of small lilac flowers. It may be propagated by seed or by cutting, and does best in full sun in a light, well-drained soil kept moist by regular watering.

PROPERTIES. Vervain contains a type of tannin peculiar to itself. Herbalists employ the whole herb including the root as a tonic, an astringent, an expectorant, a diaphoretic, and a febrifuge. It is also said to be useful for curing headaches, ophthalmia, and pleurisy and to aid nursing mothers in stimulating the flow of milk.

HOW TO USE IT.
Vervain Infusion

To compose a tonic, febrifuge, and expectorant, infuse 2 teaspoons dried vervain tops and leaves in 1 pint boiling water. Cover closely for 15 minutes before straining and flavoring with honey to taste. Allow the infusion to cool, and take 2 or 3 teaspoons 6 times a day.

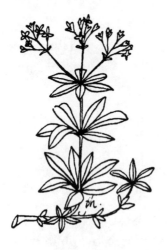

WOODRUFF
Asperula odorata

OTHER NAMES. Master of the wood. Wood-rova. Wuderove. *Muge-de-boys.* Sweet woodruff. *Waldmeister.*

HABITAT. Woodruff grows in woods and under shady hedges throughout Europe, the British Isles, and the United States. It can be recognized by its small white flowers set on slender stalks above "ruffs," or starlike groups of bright green leaves. As its old French name muge-de-boys (wood musk) implies, woodruff carries a distinctive perfume. It is derived from the presence of a chemical known to pharmacists as coumarin. Fresh sprigs of woodruff are steeped in Rhine wine to produce the fine and aromatic May wines of Germany traditionally drunk on the first of May, the old pagan festival of Beltane. The herb was also hung in aromatic bunches with roses, box, and lavender in medieval churches on the feasts of St. Peter and St. Barnabas, and its leaves are still used in some brands of herbal snuff. Woodruff is a perennial that rarely grows above 12 inches tall; it is also one of the few herbs that require full shade, so bear both of these facts in mind when you plant it. It may be grown from seed or by root division in spring or fall. Give it a good, rich earth to grow in, with regular watering.

PROPERTIES. Woodruff contains citric acid, tannin, and coumarin, an aromatic largely employed by pharmacists as a perfumery fixative, or simply to mask unpleasant odors in preparations, like that of iodoform. In dried form the herb retains the scent of new-mown hay, which lingers for years, making it a valuable ingredient for linen sachets. An infusion of the dried leaves makes a fragrant and stimulating tea, while the fresh leaves crushed and laid on bruises and minor abrasions have long been said to be healing and soothing.

HOW TO USE IT.

Woodruff Tea

Infuse 1 teaspoon dried woodruff leaves in 1 covered cup boiling water for 15 minutes. Strain and sweeten with honey to taste. Take after and between meals.

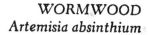

WORMWOOD
Artemisia absinthium

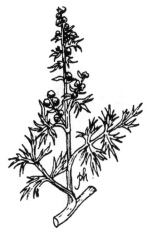

OTHER NAMES. Absinthe. Green ginger. Old woman.

HABITAT. Wormwood grows wild throughout Siberia, Europe, and the United States. In the British Isles it tends to be confined to coastal regions. It is a close relative of the mugwort (*Artemisia vulgaris*) and southernwood (*Artemisia abrotanum*). Apuleius in his herbarium informs us that Artemis, the Greek goddess of the moon and the wildwood, called Diana by the Romans, bestowed the herb upon Chiron the centaur for his healing prac-

tices. He, not unreasonably, named it Artemisia after her in grati-
tude. During the Middle Ages wormwood was considered to be an
excellent demonofuge. Witches and cunning-men made use of it in
their magic spells at every opportunity, and wreaths of it known as
St. John's girdles used to be ritually burned in the big outdoor
Midsummer fires on St. John's Eve, June 24. Wormwood's root is
perennial, and the branching stems become woody as they grow
older and may reach a height of 3 feet. The leaves are serrated,
whitish in color, and covered with fine silky hair like the stems.
They give off a bitter smell when crushed. The flowers are tiny,
green-yellow globules which appear during the summer months.
The herb may be cultivated from seed in the fall, or by cuttings, or
by root division in the fall or spring. Wormwood is a particularly
accommodating as well as attractive herb to grow, for it flourishes in
either sun or shade, and takes to any type of soil.

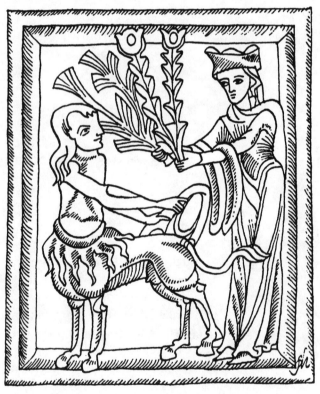

CHIRON RECEIVES WORMWOOD FROM ARTEMIS (after an Anglo-Saxon herbal)

PROPERTIES. Wormwood yields a strongly bitter essential oil which contains a variety of principles, notably thujone, phellandrine, and purine. Absinthine, tannin, some resin, and an assortment of mineral salts, including potassium nitrate, are also present. The herb's action is tonic, digestive, febrifuge, and vermifuge.

HOW TO USE IT.

Wormwood Tea

Wormwood is strongly stimulant and, taken in excessive doses, can produce vertigo and convulsions. It should therefore be used with discretion and caution. It does, however, have a built-in safety factor of sorts for many people in that it is an intensely bitter herb and more than the usual herb dose is rather disgusting!

Infuse 1 ounce dried wormwood leaves, flowers, and tops in 1 pint boiling water. Cover closely for 10 minutes before straining. Sweetening with honey or sugar is a must for most people. Take by wineglass doses up to but not exceeding 1 cup per day.

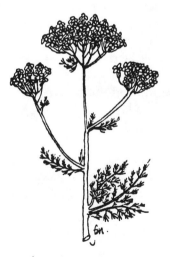

YARROW
Achillea millefolium

OTHER NAMES. Milfoil. Thousand seal. Nosebleed. Old man's pepper. Soldier's woundwort. *Herbe militaris.* Carpenter's weed. Bloodwort. Staunchweed. Sanguinary. Devil's nettle. Devil's plaything. Bad man's plaything. Yarroway. Gearwe.

HABITAT. Yarrow grows wild throughout the world, thriving in grass meadows, in waste land, and at roadsides. Gardeners consider the wild variety a troublesome weed, especially when it finds its way into the lawn. However, garden varieties are cultivated as summer- and fall-blooming perennials.

The name "yarrow" derives from the Anglo-Saxon *gearwe.* The Latin name is more informative, however. *Achillea* refers to the

Greek hero Achilles, who during the Trojan Wars was said to have staunched the wounds of his soldiers with this herb. "Bloodwort," "staunchweed," and "sanguinary" also point to this usage. *Millefolium* simply means "thousand leaves," and you will see how accurate a name this is when you take a look at the plant. The intriguing "bad man's plaything" and the various "devil's" names refer to yarrow's potential as a witch's herb, about which we shall have more to say in a later chapter.

Yarrow grows with a straight sectionally angular stem bearing alternate gray-green feathery, finely divided leaves. The dried stems are still employed by Chinese fortunetellers to consult an ancient book of oracular wisdom known as the *I Ching*, or *Book of Changes*. Carl Jung, the pioneer depth psychologist, recently introduced the *I Ching* to the West as a device for psychological introspection, but in today's popular usage the oracle is consulted by means of permutations made by three tossed coins rather than the traditional fifty yarrow sticks.

Stalk, flowers, and leaves give off a bitter fragrance when crushed. Yarrow can grow as high as 5 feet, although its more usual height is between 6 and 12 inches. It springs up in clumps, which should be divided every other year to prevent crowding. It requires full sun, regular soil, and only moderate watering. The tall flowering stems should be cut back to ensure healthy growth after they have finished blooming.

PROPERTIES. Yarrow contains an essential oil, an active component known as achillein, tannin, resin, mucilage, and a selection of mineral salts. Herbalists use it as an astringent, a tonic, a stimulant, an aromatic, and a diaphoretic.

How TO USE IT.

Mrs. Grieve considered yarrow tea an excellent remedy for severe colds and fevers. Stronger doses extracted by decoction have been used as a lotion for burns and as a specific for hemorrhoids and kidney disorders, for the astringent quality of the herb gives it definite blood-staunching capabilities.

Yarrow Tea

Infuse 1 teaspoon dried yarrow leaves and flowers in 1 covered cup boiling water for 10 minutes. Strain and sweeten with honey to taste. Drink warm between meals at the onset of fever or chill as often as required.

A more complex and potent blend may be composed as follows:
Yarrow Blend Tea

To compose a diaphoretic febrifuge, mix equal portions of yarrow, pennyroyal, catnip, spearmint, sage, verbena, and horehound. Infuse 1 teaspoon in 1 covered cup boiling water for 10 minutes. Strain and flavor with honey if required. Drink warm every 4 hours, or more frequently if more sweating is needed.

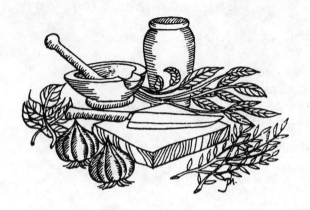

2

HERBS TO COOK WITH

THE MOST WIDELY RECOGNIZED USE FOR herbs today is in cooking; they have been used for this since the time of the ancient Egyptians. Though not a vital adjunct to rudimentary cooking of the sort that simply holds body and soul together, herbs do assume considerable importance when people begin to cultivate their sense of taste. Only through herbs can the subtler nuances of flavor be achieved. However, strange to say, this use of herbs within the kitchen, though as old as history itself, is only now beginning to catch the public fancy after several decades in abeyance. Many people, in England, for instance, to their own disadvantage, have held until quite recently that there was something slightly strange and "foreign" about using herbs in cooking. Such an attitude is, of course, ridiculous. Cooking with herbs is the only way to cook. All the best chefs—and I use the word "all" unqualifiedly—all the greatest cooks past and present have used herbs in their dishes.

During the seventeenth and eighteenth centuries, when European cookery first began to emerge as a fine art, all vegetables were known broadly as herbs. Those we would know today as table vegetables were called pot-herbs. This category included any leaves and roots that had to be cooked, such as cabbages, broccoli, spinach, turnips, and so on. Then there were the salad herbs, vegetables eaten raw, like lettuce, cress, and escarole. Lastly there were the sweet herbs, plants used not in bulk but in small amounts for flavoring and seasoning—what today we call kitchen herbs. Though the amounts in which these sweet herbs are used in cooking are considerably smaller than those for medicinal purposes, the herbs themselves are all old friends of ours from Chapter 1. We are simply making use of their most important, and least hidden property: their essential oil. All sweet herbs contain essential oils. An essential oil, without going into abstruse chemical definitions, is simply an organically produced, volatile (that is, quickly evaporating) oil produced by a plant, containing not only an active (drug) principle but often, because of its volatility, a strong aroma too. The oil is produced in tiny glands within the plant. When you "season" a dish with a certain herb, you are mingling the essential oil with the food. It may "taste" different to you, but actually the aroma is perceived more at the back of the nose than with the taste buds on the tongue, although it does affect them too. Essential oil-producing herbs that you can grow in your garden may generally speaking be divided into one or other of the two big plant families we ran across in Chapter 1: the Umbelliferae, umbrella-flower plants sometimes known generically as the hemlocks; and the Labiatae, or deadnettles, so-called lipped plants, again with reference to the flowers.

There are five lesser families which also contain valuable herbs: the "Compositae" (many-petaled, like the dandelion and tarragon), the Rutaceae (e.g., rue), the Boraginaceae (e.g., borage), the Rosaceae (e.g., the rose and burnet), and the Lauraceae (e.g., the bay laurel). However, by far the majority of kitchen herbs are contained within the hemlocks and deadnettles. The kitchen "spices" are another matter altogether, being mostly derived from exotic Middle and Far Eastern plant families. These are still herbs, however, and their value lies entirely in their essential oils.

Setting Up Your Kitchen Herb Cabinet

YOUR BASIC HERBS

The Umbelliferae

If you grow them yourself you will note that the Umbelliferae possess hollow, cylindrical stems, and compound (that is, deeply indented, as opposed to merely notched) leaves arranged alternately upon their stems. Their flowers are small and spread out in umbrellalike clusters. Their essential oil is generally concentrated in their *seeds*.

Useful kitchen Umbelliferae are:

COMMON NAME	LATIN NAME
Anise (seeds)	*Pimpinella anisum*
Caraway or kümmel (seeds)	*Carum carvi*
Celery (seeds)	*Apium graveolens*
Chervil (leaves)	*Anthriscus cerefolium*
Coriander (leaves)	*Coriandrum sativum*
Cumin (seeds)	*Cuminum cyminum*
Dill (seeds and leaves)	*Anethum graveolens*
Fennel (seeds and leaves)	*Foeniculum vulgare*
Lovage (leaves)	*Levisticum officinale*
Parsley (seeds and leaves)	*Carum petroselinum*

The Labiatae

The Labiatae possess sectionally square stems, and flowers that grow out of the intersection between leaves and stem. Often the flowers form entire tiers, or whorls, around the stem, which generally tapers to a flower-clad spike. The all-important oil glands are contained within the *leaves*.

Useful kitchen Labiatae are:

Common Name	Latin Name
Basil (leaves)	*Ocimum basilicum*
Marjoram (leaves)	*Origanum marjorana*
Oregano (leaves)	*Origanum vulgare*
Rosemary (leaves)	*Rosmarinus officinalis*
Sage (leaves)	*Salvia officinalis*
Savory, summer (leaves)	*Satureia hortensis*
Savory, winter (leaves)	*Satureia montana*
Spearmint (leaves)	*Mentha viridis*
Thyme (leaves)	*Thymus vulgaris*

If you plan to use fresh herbs grown from your own garden or planter in your cooking, the rule to remember is to use twice as much fresh, green herb as you would the dried variety. When an herb dries, it shrivels and contracts in size and weight, although the amount of all-important essential oil remains the same. Never underestimate the power of dried herbs. A small pinch may look pretty puny, but don't you believe it. Err on underdoing the herb rather than the reverse.

The practice of flavoring food with herbs is a genuine and inventive art. As such, there are no absolute rules to follow, for who is to dictate taste to anyone? But for the beginner there are a few generally held guidelines that have been evolved by centuries of trial and error. Certain herbs *do*, in the consensus of opinion, seem to complement and bring out the flavor of certain foods: fennel and fish, for one example; tarragon and chicken, for another.

The nineteen Umbelliferae and Labiatae we have just examined plus one Composita, one Liliacea, and one Lauracea—namely, tarragon, chives, and bay—are your twenty-two basic kitchen herbs. Most grocery stores and supermarkets stock all of them in dried form if you don't plan on growing them. If you have difficulty in obtaining lovage, and don't grow it yourself, try your nearest specialty-food store, or, failing that, simply send off to your handy mail-order company. The latter is by far the cheapest way, in any event, for you do not end up paying for a fancy container and label, which accounts for 50 per cent of the retail cost.

YOUR BASIC SPICES

There is no hard and fast distinction between spices and herbs. As we have already noted, they are definitely herbs, too, albeit for the most part exotic ones. However, generally speaking, a spice consists of a seed, root, flower, or fruit rather than a leaf. Some cooks therefore categorize all the Umbelliferae as spices. Spices are without exception much more powerful than leaf herbs, and whereas the latter have to be used with discretion, spices have to be used with definite caution! You can get away with an overherbed dish, but too much spice completely kills the original flavor of the food.

Your basic kitchen spices are the following:

COMMON NAMES	LATIN NAMES
Allspice; Jamaica pepper; pimento (fruit)	*Pimenta officinalis*
Cardamom; Cardamon (fruit)	*Elettaria cardamomum,* among others
Cayenne pepper; chili pepper (fruit)	*Capsicum minimum*
Cinnamon (bark)	*Laurus cinnamomum; Cinnamomum zeylanicum,* among others
Cloves (flowers)	*Eugenia aromatica,* among others
Coriander (the fruit this time)	*Coriandrum sativum*
Ginger (root)	*Zingiber officinale*
Juniper (berries)	*Juniperus communis*
Mace (outer casing of the nutmeg)	*Myristica officinalis,* among others
Mustard (seeds)	Cruciferae family
Nutmeg (fruit)	*Myristica officinalis,* among others
Paprika; Hungarian pepper (fruit)	*Croton annum*
Pepper, black and white (fruit)	Piperaceae family

COMMON NAMES	LATIN NAMES
Poppy seed (seeds)	*Papaver rhoeas*
Saffron (flowers)	*Crocus sativus*
Sesame (seeds)	Sesamum family
Vanilla beans (fruit pods)	*Vanilla aromatica,*
	among others

How to Use Your Herbs and Spices

There are, of course, endless variations upon the uses of herbs and spices in cookery. Every cook has his or her own specialties. In the following section I have tried to give a broad indication of what type of food the particular herb or spice has always been considered best suited to, and to give a demonstration recipe or two (most are staunchly nonmacrobiotic) for which I can vouch as being both simple and delicious. All cookbooks list the spices needed in their recipes, but my aim has been to approach the subject from the other way round. Given the herb or spice, especially if it happens to grow in your garden or planter, what can you *do* with it? Well, you must above all be inventive, but your inventiveness should at first be based on those cookery guidelines mentioned earlier. Once you have built up your taste vocabulary, you have earned your wings and can feel free to try soaring into the realms of exotic herbs, like sorrel, yarrow, or wormwood. But for now let's start with your basics. You may be surprised at the number of uses you can put them to.

ALLSPICE

In England, the allspice container is usually trotted out at Yule for Christmas puddings, and then shoved to the back of the shelf for the remainder of the year. This is a shame, because allspice is a remarkably versatile spice and deserves to be used more than it is. Its taste, as its name indicates, suggests a blend of cloves, nutmeg, and cinnamon, and it will lend a fragrant and distinctive flavor to any syrup you make out of wine and sugar in which you plan to simmer fruit. (Try Pears Bordelaise with allspice instead of cinnamon; see under Cinnamon.) However, its use in desserts is dwarfed by its many applications to savory dishes. For instance, try adding 3 or 4 whole allspice seeds to the water when you poach fish or boil shrimp. Similarly, fried chicken, meat stew, casserole, or pea soup will benefit enormously from the addition of 4 or 5 whole seeds. Pea soup is particularly delicious with allspice.

Split-pea Soup with Allspice

¼ cup cubed salt pork
1 cup chopped celery
1 cup chopped onion
2 teaspoons salt
1 pound split peas,
    soaked overnight and drained

1 ham hock
1 bay leaf
1 tablespoon chopped
    parsley
5 allspice seeds

Brown the salt pork in a large kettle for 5 minutes, and add the celery, onion, and salt. Cook until tender, then add 2½ quarts cold water, the soaked split peas, the ham hock, and the spices tied up in a cheesecloth bag. Bring slowly to a boil, and simmer gently for 2 hours. Remove the ham hock and the spices. Strip the meat off the bone, returning it to the soup, but discarding the bone and cheesecloth bag. Sliced frankfurter or Polish sausage may be added to the soup before serving. This soup serves 6 to 8 persons, and is really a meal in itself, especially when served with a crusty loaf of French bread.

ANISE

Anise may be used in pickling, in cream cheeses, and to enhance the flavor of certain seafoods, notably shellfish, cod, crab, and shrimp. However, its chief use in European cooking is to add zing to baked goods, confections, and fruit compotes.

A dead easy and really delicious example of anise bakery can be made as follows:

Continental Anise Cookies

12 eggs
3½ cups white sugar
4 cups sifted flour

1¼ cups cornstarch
¼ cup anise seed

Beat the eggs and sugar together and blend in the flour, cornstarch, and anise. Make macaroon-sized drops upon a moistened cookie sheet, and leave in a warm place until the drops begin to rise. Bake in a medium (350°) oven until the cookies are golden brown.

BASIL

Basil is one of the most widely used herbs in Mediterranean cookery. It may be introduced to any egg dish with excellent results, and adds wonderful dimension to any bouillabaisse or fish chowder, as well as to baked, poached, or broiled fish of any type. Tomatoes and eggplants respond extremely well to a basil garnish or stuffing, especially if you are lucky enough to have the fresh herb on hand. Spaghetti or linguine also goes fabulously with a basil sauce, or pesto.

Nina Foch gave me this recipe, and I must say it beats any in the regular cookbooks.

Pesto Genovese

½ cup pine nuts, coarsely grated
½ cup freshly grated Parmesan cheese
½ cup whipped butter, at room temperature
4 large peeled cloves garlic (no reticence here)
1 teaspoon salt
¼ cup olive oil
1 pinch cayenne
1 cup fresh basil leaves, washed, stripped
    from their stems, and firmly packed
1 tablespoon water if needed
A few leaves of fresh marjoram,
    washed and dried (optional)

Mix the pine nuts, cheese, and butter well by hand in a bowl. In an electric blender place the garlic, salt, oil, and cayenne, and blend thoroughly. Introduce the basil leaves slowly, and blend to a smooth, green, fragrant paste! Pour this into the bowl and mix well with Parmesan-pine .nuts, and *eccò!* Pesto Genovese! Simply toss the hot spaghetti or linguine in it until well coated before serving. For those who prefer a blander mixture, add a little ricotta cheese to the pesto before tossing in your pasta.

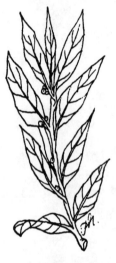

BAY

Bay trees or bushes make very attractive additions to any garden, and they are particularly handy for potting and decorating your urban rooftop bower. The leaves possess a marvelously mellow, almost regal aroma. Little wonder the Greeks and Romans used wreaths of them to crown their victorious athletes and generals. Because of their toughness, bay leaves have to be steeped in alcohol or heated before they surrender their essence. Hence they are usually employed in wine marinades (for any type of meat except pork) or added to chowders, stews, bouillons, and pilafs. Like basil, they complement the flavor of tomatoes beautifully, but the tomatoes will have to be heated first in a bouillon or sauce before the bay will work its magic.

Bay Marinade

A marinade is a sauce that resembles an herbal oil-and-wine salad dressing in which one presoaks a cut of meat before roasting or braising it. It is a particularly useful device to employ if the meat is not a very good cut or just plain tough. In fact, marinating is really the only sure way of making tough meat palatable without using tenderizer. The following marinade may be used with lamb, veal, or beef, whether the meat is in a whole roast or cut up in chops or shishkebab-type chunks.

¾ cup red wine	1 pinch ground black pepper
¼ cup olive oil	1 bay leaf, crumbled
3 cloves garlic, crushed	½ teaspoon thyme (optional)
1 teaspoon salt	½ teaspoon marjoram (optional)

Mix the ingredients together in a large bowl, and marinate the meat in it, turning it every so often to ensure complete immersion, for *at least* 1 hour, preferably longer, before broiling, pot-roasting, or roasting on a rack. The tougher the cut of meat, the longer you should marinate it. For periods longer than a day, keep the meat marinating in the refrigerator.

CARAWAY SEEDS

Caraway, or kümmel, as it is known on the Continent, like anise, is used chiefly to flavor pickles, cheeses, and bakery goods. However, it can also be used to great advantage to enhance the taste of any cabbage dish. Try sprinkling a pinch of caraway seeds in your cole slaw and see the difference. Or try this:

Buttered Cabbage with Caraway

Wash, core, and cut your cabbage into wedges or shreds. Cook in a covered pan in a *small* amount of boiling water until *just* tender. Do not overcook. Drain well and season with salt, a pinch of black pepper, and a small pinch of caraway seeds. Then serve with a tablespoonful of butter.

CARDAMOM

Cardamom is one of the few spices which is used almost exclusively in sweet dishes. The pale round pods contain tiny black seeds. Both pod and seed are highly perfumed, and make a powerful ingredient in any sachet mixture (see Chapter 3). Cardamom also makes a fabulous addition to any spiced wine or hippocras (see p. 175ff.), and 1 or 2 crushed pods will transform your evening pot of coffee into gorgeously scented "Arabian coffee." Cardamom seeds may be added with impunity to any jelly or fruit compote. They also do wonders to any home-made jam. I have a wretched Seville orange tree in my garden which produces the most vile, bitter-tasting fruit. However, with the alchemy of a few cloves and cardamom seeds I have found that the oranges can be transformed into the most fragrant and delicious marmalade.

Cardamom Orange Marmalade

Wash the oranges and slice them thinly. Add 1½ times their volume of water, and 3 cloves, crushed, and 3 cardamoms, crushed, for each quart of liquid. Let stand overnight, and cook slowly the following day until the peel is tender (2 to 2½ hours). Measure the quantity to which your marmalade has boiled down, and add ⅔ to equal the *volume* of white sugar, depending on the sweetness desired. Bring back to a boil, and cook briskly until the marmalade jells on a wooden spoon (50 to 60 minutes).

CAYENNE

Cayenne, or chili, pepper is really the fruit of the capsicum pepper, a plant from the same family as the tomato and the deadly nightshade, and a native of India. The words "cayenne" and "capsicum" both come from the Greek meaning "to bite," and this is quite a fair assessment of the spice's action. Although, strange to say, it is useful in herbal medicine as a digestive aid, cayenne employed in cooking needs to be used only in the smallest amounts, unless one relishes hot food or has a mouth with a cast-iron lining. In northern European cooking it is used chiefly in sauces, pickles, salad dressings, egg dishes, and cheese dips. It is, however, an indispensable ingredient of many curry powders and most Mexican dishes. chili con carne, for instance:

Easy Chili con Carne

1 onion, chopped	½ teaspoon celery seed
3 cloves garlic, finely chopped	¼ teaspoon crushed cumin seed
3 tablespoons olive oil	1 bay leaf
1 pound chopped or ground beef	2 tablespoons chili powder
1½ cups canned tomatoes	¼ teaspoon basil
1 green pepper, chopped	1½ teaspoons salt

Brown the onion and garlic in the oil in a large pan, then add the ground beef. Brown well before tossing in the other ingredients. Stir well, bring to a boil, and simmer for 3 hours. For chili and beans, mix in a can of kidney beans 10 minutes before serving.

Homemade Curry Powder

To be used on any meat curry, in mayonnaise, baked beans, soups, rice, or hashes.

1½ teaspoons crushed caraway seed
1½ teaspoons crushed coriander seed
1½ teaspoons crushed cumin seed
¾ teaspoon ground ginger root
¾ teaspoon ground black pepper
½ teaspoon crushed cardamom seed
¼ teaspoon ground nutmeg
¼ teaspoon dry mustard
¼ teaspoon ground cloves
¼ teaspoon cayenne pepper

One and a half teaspoons turmeric, or fenugreek seeds obtainable from your local gourmet shop, may be substituted for the caraway if a really authentic Indian flavor is desired.

CELERY SEED

Celery seed gives a dish exactly the same flavor as celery stalk and root. The seed is just more convenient to have on hand. It may be used in cheese dishes, seafood, vegetable juices, any type of salad, stewed tomatoes, potatoes, eggplant, and cabbage. Meatloaf, stew, and meat stuffing also benefit enormously from the addition of a little celery seed. It is one of the important ingredients in many of the bouquets garnis of French haute cuisine.

Bouquet Garni I

For use in any stew, stock, or casserole where a delicate seasoning is required:

> 1 pinch celery seed
> 1 large pinch tarragon
> 1 sprig fresh parsley
> 1 large pinch chervil
> 6 whole black peppercorns

Tie the herbs up in a piece of washed cheesecloth and place the bag in your casserole or pot of stew while it cooks. Remove before serving. If you make the string tying the cheesecloth long enough to hang over the side of the pot, this will facilitate its removal.

See also Bouquet Garni II on p. 125.

CHERVIL

Chervil is a close relative of parsley, although its flavor is infinitely more refined. The flavor is so subtle, in fact, that cooks generally find that it needs to be blended with the flavor of other herbs to really work. You will find that chervil, tarragon, chives, and basil complement one another well. Chervil can be used in salads, green vegetables (broccoli, spinach, peas, or asparagus), cream cheeses, and dips. It also works wonders with egg dishes of any type. Try it and you'll see what I mean.

Eggs with Chervil

6 eggs
2 tablespoons butter
2 tablespoons heavy cream
1 teaspoon chopped chives
  or scallions

1 large pinch chervil
1 large pinch tarragon
  (optional)
Black pepper and salt to taste

Beat the eggs until well mixed, and pour them into a pan in which the butter has been melted over a low heat. Cook slowly, stirring all the while, until the eggs begin to set. Add the cream, chives, herbs and seasonings, and continue cooking until the desired consistency is achieved.

CHIVES

The chive comes from the same plant family as the garlic, the leek, and the onion. It is a refined cousin of the scallion, or spring onion. Chopped chive tops make a delicious addition to omelets, egg dishes, and any sauce that requires a subtle onionlike flavor. They should not be cooked long, but should rather be added at the end of the cooking. Combined with a dollop of sour cream, they make an excellent and time-honored garnish for baked potatoes.

Chive Butter

2 tablespoons chopped fresh chives
1 pound butter
1 pinch salt (optional)

Bring the butter to room temperature, and whip in the chives and salt. Refrigerate and serve with hot rolls, hot biscuits, or baked potatoes.

Other herbed butters you can try are rosemary, to accompany

lamb, steak, or fish; tarragon for chicken; oregano for grilled tomatoes; and chervil for egg dishes and omelets. All herbed butters should be used within 8 days.

CINNAMON

Cinnamon bark, like cardamom, is a spice, used chiefly in sweet dishes, jams, jellies, and fruits, although in Eastern and Middle Eastern dishes it appears quite frequently in meat recipes. It can be used to enliven any drab milk pudding or custard and, again like cardamom, will add an exciting new flavor to your coffee. Baked apples taste fabulous when cored and filled with a mixture of brown sugar, a dab of butter, raisins, a clove, and a pinch of cinnamon before being popped in a medium oven for 40 minutes or so. Any type of syrup for stewing fruit such as the one which follows can be flavored with cinnamon.

Pears Bordelaise

4 to 6 pears
½ cup red wine
1 cup white sugar
½ lemon
1 stick cinnamon (you can use cinnamon powder, but
   it makes the mixture muddy)

Peel, core, and halve the pears. Combine the wine, sugar, the lemon half (squeezed), both peel and juice, and the cinnamon stick in a pan and bring to the boil, stirring gently. Introduce the pear halves 2 at a time if your pan is a small one, until all the pears are tender. Reduce the remaining liquor until it reaches a syrupy consistency and pour it over the pears. Chill and serve. Serves 4 to 6 persons, depending on how greedy they are.

CLOVES

Cloves are used in both savory and sweet dishes. They can be added in ground form to plum pudding, or whole to any cooked fruit, jam, jelly, mulled wine, hot tea, or even hot chocolate. When using them whole, you can tie them up in a cheesecloth bag for easy removal. Apropos savory dishes, cloves can be added to the cooking water of beets, carrots, or squash. They are a must with sweet potatoes. Any type of stock, especially if you make it with an onion floating in it, does well with the addition of a couple of cloves. Baked ham is particularly delicious with them:

Home-baked Ham with Cloves

> 1 uncooked ham
> 12 to 18 whole cloves
> 1 cup brown sugar
> 2 teaspoons mustard powder

Preheat oven to 300° F. Wash ham rind well, dry, and bake until a meat thermometer registers 160°—about 25 minutes per pound. Remove ham from oven, cut off the rind, and score the underlying fat diagonally with a sharp knife in diamond pattern. (You can do a crisscross one if you prefer, but diamonds are traditional.) Insert the sharp ends of the cloves in the corners of the diamonds, and then coat the entire surface of the fat with a mixture of a little fat from your pan and the sugar and mustard. Turn up the oven to 400° F., and bake the ham once more until the sugar has formed a glaze.

CORIANDER

Both the seeds and the leaves of the coriander are used in cooking. The seeds are readily available at your local grocery, but to obtain the leaves without growing them yourself may lead you to visit your nearest Italian or Spanish produce store, where they appear under the name of cilentro or culantro respectively. Some mail-order companies handle them, too. The seeds find a use in curry powders, meatloafs, pork roasts, gravies, and certain desserts. The leaves, however, to my mind a particularly exotic delicacy, are generally used only in Mexican or Italian cooking. They are a primary ingredient in a savory and really delicious Mexican soup known as albondigas, which is well worth making if you like meatballs.

Albondigas Soup

1 slice white bread
½ pound lean ground pork
1 pound lean ground beef
1 egg
1 clove garlic, finely chopped
1 pinch sage
1 pinch spearmint

⅛ teaspoon chopped fresh culantro
1 pinch black pepper
1 teaspoon salt
1 onion, chopped
2 tablespoons fat or cooking oil
1 tomato, mashed

Soak the bread in water, squeeze it out, and mix it in well with the pork and beef. Add the egg, garlic, herbs, and seasonings; mold into walnut-sized meatballs. Brown the onion in the fat or oil, and remove from the pan. Brown the meatballs, and when they are good and fried, reintroduce the onion, the tomato, and 4 to 6 cups boiling water. Bring to a boil and simmer for 1½ hours before serving. Serves 4 to 6.

CUMIN

Cumin, as we have seen, comes from the same plant family as anise and caraway, and can be used in almost exactly the same way. However, whereas anise and caraway have a comparatively delicate flavor, cumin has a rather aggressive one. Like coriander, cumin constitutes one of the ingredients of curry powder, and is also used largely in Mexican and Italian dishes. If you have ever shopped in a Spanish or Italian food market, you will recognize its smell immediately.

Cumin seeds may be used to spike up any cheese dip or savory sandwich spread with great effect. Some cooks use it in fruit tarts and pies, but many find the taste rather too dominant for sweets. Chili and curry dishes, plus any type of pilaf or *arroz con pollo*, will benefit enormously from the addition of a pinch of bruised cumin seed.

Chicken Pilaf with Cumin

½ cup butter
2 cups long-grain rice
1 quart hot chicken broth
Salt and pepper to taste
Cumin seed

Melt the butter in a deep pan and brown the rice, stirring continuously, for 5 minutes. Add the broth, seasonings, and cumin; stir. Cover and simmer gently until the rice has absorbed all the liquid.

DILL

Dill is sold in both seed and leaf form, the former being more powerful than the latter. It is used for flavoring any number of different vegetables, cocktail dips, pickles, fish, and some meats, notably lamb. It is really most valuable in vegetables and salads, however. Cabbage, cucumber, beet, lettuce, potato, and seafood salads do well with a little dill weed sprinkled on them. Cooked beets, broccoli, brussels sprouts, cabbage, green beans, and turnips also improve considerably with a pinch of dill in melted butter poured over them after cooking. For cucumber salads dill is a must.

Cucumber in Dill Sauce

1 cucumber
½ onion
½ pint sour cream
1 good pinch dill weed
Salt and white pepper to taste

Wash and peel the cucumber, slice it thin, and press it between paper towels to remove some of the excess liquid. Grate the onion and mix it with the sour cream, dill weed, and sliced cucumber. Season to taste with salt and pepper. Chill for at least 1 day before serving.

A Quaint, but Perfectly Usable "Dill and Collyflower [Cauliflower] Pickle" [1]

"Boil the Collyflowers till they fall in pieces; then with some of the stalk and worst of the flower boil it in a part of the liquer till pretty strong. Then being taken off strain it, and when settled, clean it from the bottom. Then with Dill, gross [whole] pepper, a pretty quantity of salt, when cold add as much vinegar as will make it sharp and pour all upon the Collyflower."

FENNEL

Fennel seed, like that of all the other Umbelliferae, may be sprinkled on top of bread and rolls before baking. It also goes well

[1] From *Acetaria, a Book about Sallets*, by John Evelyn (1680).

with rice dishes, cream cheeses, and bland Italian cheeses such as mozzarella. Chicken, beef, pork, and lamb, but especially pork, taste marvelous if rubbed with a little bruised fennel seed and garlic before roasting. Try it in sausage meat too. However, fennel's virtue really appears when it is combined with any fish, particularly an oily one, such as tuna. Here is my own recipe for what I consider a delicious tuna salad:

Tuna Salad

1 stick celery	1 large pinch thyme
6 scallions	1 large pinch chervil
8 tablespoons real mayonnaise	1 large pinch fennel seed
1 pound canned tuna (chunk style)	6 black peppercorns

Wash and trim the celery and scallions, removing all of the latter except for the white ends and a small portion of the stalks. Chop them finely and combine in a bowl with the mayonnaise and tuna. Pound the herbs and the peppercorns in a pestle and mortar and add mixture to the tuna. Toss well, and serve on young leaves of fresh, crunchy lettuce.

Fines Herbes for Any Fish

Take equal parts of marjoram, sage, basil, thyme, bruised fennel seed, and parsley. Combine well and sprinkle a pinch or two of the mixture on the fish before cooking.

GARLIC

Garlic may be used in moderation in any savory dish. Fresh garlic bulb is best, but it can also be obtained in powdered form, although the powder is usually frowned on by cooks who take their art really seriously.

Garlic is employed in a great many French dishes, and nearly all Mediterranean ones. It is an essential ingredient of the garlic butter used to cook snails and shrimps in. A clove or two of garlic mashed up in room-temperature butter with a little chopped fresh parsley and a pinch of oregano, if you're feeling particularly Provençal, is all there is to it. Try spreading it on a split loaf of French bread with a little Parmesan cheese sprinkled on top and toasted for 3 minutes. It's unbelievably good.

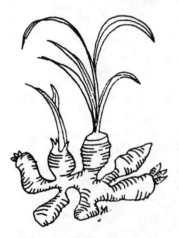

GINGER ROOT

Ginger root is a gnarled, potatolike tuber, brown on the outside, creamy yellow within. Most groceries stock the dried powdered variety. To buy it whole you may have to search out a gourmet food store, or write to one of the addresses listed at the back of the book.

Ginger is a favorite meat herb in Chinese cooking. In European dishes, however, its hot, spicy taste is reserved chiefly for stewed fruits, preserves, beers (see section on herb beers), and steamed puddings. Some chefs also use it to flavor chicken, beef, lamb, or veal stocks. If you buy it whole, which incidentally is the best way as the powdered variety loses its strength fairly rapidly, scrape off the outside brown skin before slicing and mincing it. A piece of ginger root can be tied up in a cheesecloth bag with some allspice, cloves, and stick cinnamon to provide a more complex variation of your "Bordelaise" fruit syrup.

Chinese Braised Chicken with Ginger

1 frying chicken, peeled, boned, and chopped in 2-inch pieces
Fresh ginger root
½ cup cooking oil
½ teaspoon salt
¼ teaspoon ground black pepper

Dry the chicken thoroughly with paper towels before frying. Peel and chop ginger root in enough ½-inch slices to fill ¼ cup. Heat the cooking oil in a heavy skillet until smoking, and brown the chicken and ginger root rapidly in it. Add salt and pepper, reduce the heat to medium, cover, and cook until the chicken is tender —about 30 minutes. Discard the ginger and pour off the oil before serving with rice or steamed vegetables.

JUNIPER BERRIES

Juniper is a small, shrubby conifer that grows wild in chalky soil all over Europe, Asia, North America, and North Africa. The berries contain both a resin and an essential oil, and in addition to their use in cooking and herbal medicine, they also provide the primary flavoring ingredient of gin. A close relative of the pine, the juniper possesses the same characteristic turpentine-like smell; in fact, oil of turpentine was once frequently used by less than scrupulous herb dealers as an adulterant of medicinal juniper oil.

Because of their piney tang, juniper berries give dishes a somewhat exotic flavor. Three to 5 berries, crushed, can be used to flavor any roast meat, especially game, sauerkraut (a must), dried peas or beans, lentils, squash, boiled onions, and cabbage. Soups of oxtail, beef, lamb, chicken, pea, lentil, and barley all take juniper well. Many superb French-style pâtés and terrines make excellent use of juniper berries. Here is one of them. It's unbelievably fattening, but so delicious.

William Bast's 10-minute Pâté Maison

¾ pound fat pork
¾ pound lean, cheap veal
½ pound pork liver
Butter
1 small glass sherry
1 glass white wine
1 egg, beaten

Salt and freshly ground
  black pepper to taste
2 cloves garlic, crushed
4 juniper berries, crushed
3 or 4 rashers bacon
Bouquet garni of bay, thyme,
  and parsley

Coarsely mince the pork and veal together. Fry the liver lightly in butter; remove. Add the sherry to the pan juices, cooking it until the liquid has reduced to half the original amount. Mince the liver in with the other meat, and add the wine, egg, salt, pepper, and crushed garlic and juniper berries. Mix well and turn into a terrine or breadpan. Lattice the bacon on top, place the herb bouquet upon this, and bake in a pan of water in a slow oven (325°) for 1 to 1¼ hours, covered for the first ½ hour, uncovered for the remainder. Remove herbs, cool, and serve with thin toast or crackers.

LOVAGE

Lovage comes from the same family as celery, and has a similar, though considerably stronger, yeastlike flavor. Its leaves may be used sparingly in stocks and stews, salads, mayonnaise, fish chowders, sauces, sauerkraut, and gravies. They are excellent in any soup. Try rubbing chicken or Rock Cornish game hen with a little garlic butter and lovage before roasting or broiling.

Lovage Sauce

To serve with fish, poultry or vegetables:

> 2 tablespoons butter
> 2 tablespoons flour
> 1 cup milk
> Salt and ground black pepper to taste
> 1 large pinch lovage

Melt the butter in a pan without letting it brown. Add the flour, stirring continuously with a wire whisk and cook gently for 5 minutes without browning. Bring the milk independently to the boiling point, and add it to the flour and butter, stirring briskly until the sauce thickens. Season with salt, pepper, and lovage.

MACE. See Nutmeg

MARJORAM

Marjoram and its close but rare cousin, dittany of Crete, can be used in practically any savory dish. Carrots, spinach, peas, onions, zucchini, and asparagus take its flavor well. So do chicken, duck, turkey, lamb, veal, beef, and meatloaf. Sprinkle stews with a pinch of marjoram 10 minutes before removing them from the heat. Tuna, salmon, all baked fish and shellfish improve with marjoram, as does any egg dish, omelet, or cheese dip.

Roast Beef with Marjoram

1 standing rib roast of beef
½ teaspoon salt
1 large pinch freshly ground black pepper
1 teaspoon marjoram

Preheat oven to 300° F. Moisten the roast with a damp cloth, and rub it with salt, pepper, and marjoram. Place the meat on a rack in a roasting pan and roast until done.

Rare beef—20 minutes per pound
Medium rare—22 minutes per pound
Medium—25 minutes per pound
Well done—30 minutes per pound

Marjoram Rarebit

2 teaspoons Worcestershire sauce
½ teaspoon dry mustard
1 dash paprika
1 pinch marjoram
½ cup beer
1 pound grated cheese, Cheddar

Mix all the seasonings with the beer in a pan and bring it to a boil. Then add the cheese, stirring continuously until it has melted. Serve on toast or over poached eggs.

MUSTARD

Mustard is used chiefly as a table condiment, but can be added in small quantities to sauerkraut and cole slaw to give them extra bite. It is also added to a wide variety of pickles and relishes, notably those containing beets, cucumbers, green tomatoes, cabbage, green beans, onions, and cauliflower. Most of the mustard powder obtainable in grocery stores is derived from the seeds of the white mustard plant. Black mustard seed, on the other hand, a stronger variety, is used in the condiment known as French mustard. One of mustard's most valuable uses is as an emulsifier or binder between oil and vinegar in salad dressings. Here is a trusty standby of my own invention:

Mustard Vinaigrette

A really delicious dressing for use on salads of any type.

> ½ teaspoon salt (more or less to taste)
> ¼ cup white wine vinegar
> 1 pinch monosodium glutamate (optional)
> ¼ teaspoon dry mustard
> ½ cup salad oil
> 2 cloves garlic, crushed

Mix the salt, vinegar, monosodium glutamate, and mustard together well until the mustard has completely blended. Pour in the salad oil and add the garlic. Mix thoroughly until an even consistency is achieved.

"English" Mustard (Condiment)

Simply mix dried white mustard with a little cold water until a thick, creamy consistency is achieved. To keep it from drying out too quickly in the cupboard, many people add a little cooking oil too.

A Simple "French" Mustard (Condiment)

¼ cup dried black mustard
¼ cup sugar
1½ tablespoons cornstarch
1 clove garlic, crushed (optional)

½ teaspoon salt
Up to ⅔ cup water
⅓ cup white wine vinegar

Combine the mustard, sugar, cornstarch, garlic, and salt, and add the water and vinegar slowly until a thick creamy consistency is achieved. (A little salad oil may also be added, as above.) Delicious with hot dogs or frankfurters and beans.

NUTMEG

Mace parings, or blades, as they are called, are the outside rim of the nutmeg nut. Their flavors are almost identical, but that of mace is less pungent than nutmeg. Mace is used in savory dishes, whereas the inner nutmeg itself is mostly reserved for sweet ones. Blades of mace are hard and leathery and, like bay leaves, require heating before they will surrender their flavor. When they are used in tomato juice, the juice has to be heated before being chilled and used. A couple of blades of mace may also be used in chicken or seafood sauces, soups, or stocks. Green beans, carrots, celery, onions, cauliflower, and potatoes also do well with a blade or two of mace added to their cooking water.

Nutmeg, on the other hand, in addition to the vegetables mentioned above, can be used on lima beans, corn, kale, spinach, especially sweet potatoes and squash. A dash of nutmeg is a must in all mashed potatoes. It is also delicious in any milk pudding, custard, milk drink (hot or cold), or eggnog. It complements the taste of any cooked apples or pears, and can be put to good use in both lemon and orange dessert sauces.

Old-fashioned Rice Pudding with Nutmeg

One of the easiest nutmeg recipes to make and yet one of the most tasty if you have an appetite for solid desserts is good old-fashioned rice pudding:

1 quart milk	¼ teaspoon grated nutmeg
¼ cup raw long-grain rice	½ cup raisins
½ teaspoon salt	1 teaspoon vanilla extract
½ cup white sugar	

Preheat the oven to 300° F., butter a casserole, and bake the milk, rice, salt, sugar, and nutmeg in it, uncovered, for 2 hours, stirring every ½ hour or so. While doing this, soften the raisins separately in a small amount of water, drain, add the vanilla, and mix in with the rice during the last ½ hour of baking. Serves 6 to 8.

OREGANO

Wild marjoram, or oregano, as it is now called by most cooks, is another time-honored Mediterranean standby. Most Italian dishes and many Greek, Turkish, and southern French ones will have the flavor of oregano lurking somewhere in the background. It can be used advantageously in practically any savory dish: appetizers, meats, poultry, seafood, marinades especially, stews, salads, soups, and vegetables. Go easy with it, though, for the flavor is remarkably obtrusive, and if overdone can effectively drown out the taste of what you are eating. One-eighth to ¼ teaspoon is usually enough for 4 servings. But it really is a very effective herb for conjuring up an authentic Mediterranean flavor in any dish. It goes well with all raw vegetable juices (heat and chill as with any other); rubbed on beef, lamb, veal, and pork in any form; with chicken; spaghetti sauces; shrimps, snails, and any baked fish; tomato, bean, green-pea soup, and any chowder; onions, peas, squash, tomatoes, green beans, corn, kale, and, above all, that most hard-to-flavor vegetable, spinach.

Italian Spinach

2 pounds spinach	Salt and black pepper to taste
3 tablespoons butter	Grated Parmesan cheese
3 tablespoons olive oil	1 large pinch oregano
2 cloves garlic, finely chopped (more or less as desired)	

Remove the stalks from the spinach and wash the leaves carefully, taking care to remove all sand and grit. Chop them and wilt them briefly (30 seconds) in fast-boiling salted water. Drain and set aside. Heat the butter, oil, garlic, salt, pepper, and oregano in a pan and cook slowly for 3 to 5 minutes. Add the spinach, mix thoroughly, and sprinkle the top liberally with grated cheese. Finally, set pan under a broiler to give it a crisp golden crust.

Broiled Shrimp with Oregano

The only way to eat large shrimp!

2 pounds large shrimp, shelled and deveined
½ cup olive oil
½ teaspoon salt
2 cloves garlic, finely chopped
¼ teaspoon ground black pepper
2 tablespoons chopped parsley
¼ cup butter
Juice of ½ lemon
1 large pinch oregano

Butterfly the shrimp in a baking dish; combine other ingredients and pour them over the shrimp. Bake in a hot oven (450° F.) for 10 to 12 minutes. Serve piping hot with lots of crusty French or Italian bread to soak up the sauce. Serves 4 to 6, depending on the size of the shrimp and your appetite.

PAPRIKA

Sometimes called Hungarian pepper, paprika dominates the flavor of most Hungarian goulashes. As Leonie de Sounin has aptly put it in her entertaining and informative book,[2] paprika is practically the national spice of the Balkans! It comes from the same plant family as the peppers, but its taste has none of their fierce violence. In fact, its distinctive "earthy" flavor is really quite sweet. It may be used in any savory egg dish, on meats of all kinds (before roasting or broiling), oysters, mayonnaise, fish, potatoes, salads, in any type of soup, on vegetables, and in cheese dips. One-fourth to ½ teaspoonful is usually enough for 4 servings. Incidentally, for those who are keeping an eye on the nutritional values of their seasonings, paprika is said to contain as much as five times the amount of vitamin C as lemons and oranges do.

Easy Hungarian Goulash

4 cups chopped onions
¼ cup shortening
1½ pounds stewing beef, cubed
1 small can tomato paste
1½ teaspoons salt
1 tablespoon paprika (rose or sweet)
¼ cup water

Fry the onions to a golden brown in the fat. Remove and reserve them. Fry the meat, stirring continuously for 3 minutes. Add the fried onions and other ingredients, stir well, and cover. Simmer for 1½ to 2 hours, until the meat is tender. Serve hot over noodles or rice.

[2] *Magic in Herbs* (New York: Pyramid Books, 1972).

PARSLEY

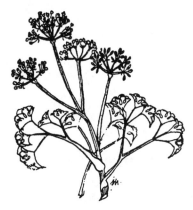

Parsley can be grown easily in any garden or planter. It does best in a well-watered soil and shady location. Although the root and seeds are used for medicinal purposes, only the leaves are used for cooking. When added to any savory dish —and they really can be added to practically any dish—they give it a marvelously fresh herby flavor, especially if they are fresh rather than dried. However, both have the same effect, the dried only a little less so than the fresh.

Parsley blends well with other herbs, and this makes it a good ingredient to put in any bouquet garni. It is a trusty standby for any egg, seafood, meat, or poultry sauce when you have nothing more exotic (like chervil or lovage) to employ. The same applies to potato and egg salads and all cooked vegetables. Any type of stew meat, poultry, or fish can have a handful of chopped fresh parsley tossed in 10 minutes before serving. Sprigs of parsley are also widely used as a tasty as well as decorative garnish for any savory dish you wish to dress up: savories and appetizers, salads, fish and seafood, roasts, poultry, and game of all sorts. When you serve soups or vegetable juices, try sprinkling a teaspoon of freshly chopped leaves on top. Like paprika, parsley has a high content of vitamin C, and also of iron.

Bouquet Garni II

For use with any stew, stock, or casserole where a more robust seasoning is required:

> 1 sprig fresh parsley
> 1 large pinch thyme
> 1 large pinch marjoram
> 1 bay leaf, crumbled

Prepare as in Bouquet Garni I (see p. 108).

Parsley Butter

For use with any cooked vegetables, but especially with potatoes and carrots:

> ½ cup butter
> 2 tablespoons chopped fresh parsley
> ½ teaspoon lemon juice
> Salt to taste

Melt the butter; mix well with the other ingredients. Toss vegetables in it before serving.

PEPPER, BLACK AND WHITE

Pepper is a hot spice berry that may be safely used on any savory dish. It comes in two varieties, "black" and "white," both derived from the same berry. Black is the stronger of the two. White pepper, the inner fruit of the peppercorn minus the hot black outer husk, is used chiefly for its esthetic effect, namely in pale foods such as white fish, or in white sauces where specks of black pepper would obtrude. It is also used in bland vegetable soups or in dishes where the flavor of pepper is required without too much of its heat. Pepper when cooked in food releases its flavor to a greater extent than when it is merely added as an afterthought, so remember—a pinch of pepper in cooking will go a long way, especially in soups. Ideally, pepper should be purchased whole and ground in a mill or a mortar just before use, for once ground it loses its kick rapidly. Pepper may be used on all meats or seafoods, in all vegetables, juices, cheese dips, and sauces, any egg dish, marinade, or soup. Add a large pinch of coarsely ground black pepper to the salt and other herbs with which you rub your roast before you place it in the oven. If you find you enjoy the flavor of pepper in and of itself, try a pepper steak. For those who appreciate hot food, they are irresistible!

Pepper Steak

2 tablespoons cooking brandy	Butter
Salt	Worcestershire sauce
Garlic	Tabasco sauce
Steaks for grilling or broiling	Lemon juice
Coarsely ground black pepper	

Set the brandy to warm on the back of the stove in a small pan. Sprinkle a thin layer of salt over the bottom of a heavy frying pan. Crush the garlic—1 clove to each steak—and spread both sides of the steaks with it. Then sprinkle the steaks liberally (¼ to ½ teaspoon each) with the pepper, pressing it in firmly with the ball of your hand. Heat the salted pan over a high flame, and when the salt begins to spit and turn brown, lay the steaks in the pan. Thirty seconds will produce a rare steak, longer for a more well-done one. Turn the meat when it has browned on one side and cook for 1 more minute. Lower the heat, lay a pat of butter on top of each steak, and add a dash of Worcestershire sauce, Tabasco, and lemon juice to taste. Turn the flame completely off now, add brandy, and (look out for your eyebrows here) apply a lighted match to burn off the alcohol. Serve and pour the pan juices over the steaks.

POPPY SEEDS

We shall be taking a closer look at the poppy in Chapter 6, when we examine some of the more recondite aspects of herb lore. Suffice it to say for now that it is the white poppy, *Papaver somniferum* that provides the spice cabinet with its seeds, not its lesser cousin the red *Papaver rhoeas*. The leaves and flowers of both varieties are narcotic, the red considerably less so than the white, although the narcotic properties are absent from the seeds. Poppy seeds are rich in an oil that has been used for centuries by artists as a drying oil to mix with paints, second only in popularity to linseed. It is also used in France as a salad oil, for it has the advantage of storing well and remaining relatively odorless. The toasted nutty-flavored seeds themselves are used mainly as a topping for cookies, breads, and rolls and in honey fillings for Hungarian coffee cakes. Noodles and most vegetables also taste delicious when buttered and lightly dusted with toasted poppy seeds. Try them in cream cheese too.

Toasted Poppy Seeds

Sprinkle the seeds over the bottom of a baking dish and toast in a 350° F. oven for 20 minutes, or heat them in a pan over a low flame on top of the stove. Use them while they are still warm.

Poppy-seed Cake Filling

½ cup crushed poppy seeds
¼ cup milk
½ cup brown sugar
2 tablespoons butter
2 egg yolks

½ cup ground almonds
2 tablespoons honey
2 teaspoons lemon juice
1 teaspoon vanilla extract

Boil the poppy seeds in the milk, and add the brown sugar and butter. Remove from the heat and stir in the egg yolks. Heat gently, stirring continuously, until a thick custard begins to form. Remove from the heat once more and add the almonds, honey, lemon juice, and vanilla.

ROSEMARY

Rosemary is a versatile and fragrant herb as useful to perfumery as it is to cooking. It may be used in any savory egg dish. Try it in scrambled eggs or omelets, as a variation from chives, chervil, basil, or tarragon. Rosemary will also bring out and complement the taste of any baked oily fish, fish stew, or casserole. Pork, lamb, beef, veal, and chicken all take the flavor of rosemary well; rub them with a little (with or without garlic) before roasting. It also tastes good in a variety of soups: potato, spinach, or pea. Even if you don't flavor your roast with rosemary, try sprinkling a few potatoes with some and roasting them alongside.

Chicken with Rosemary

1 roasting chicken	1 sprig parsley
1 tablespoon lemon juice	Freshly ground black pepper
½ teaspoon salt	1 teaspoon rosemary
1 small onion, roughly chopped	Butter
1 clove garlic, finely chopped	

Preheat oven to 350° F. Wash and dry the chicken thoroughly inside and out, and then rub the inner cavity first with the lemon juice, then with the salt. Now stuff it with the onion, garlic, parsley, black pepper, and rosemary, and fasten the cavity shut with meat skewers. Place the chicken breast up on a roasting rack in a pan, and butter it well. Roast it in the oven until it is a golden brown, basting with extra butter every 30 to 40 minutes.

SAFFRON

Saffron was once a native of the Far East, but now grows throughout Europe. Probably the most expensive common culinary spice on the market today, it is made out of the pistils of crocuses—the tiny filaments in the center of the flowers—which goes a good deal of the way toward explaining its extraordinary price. It is said to require 60,000 crocus pistils to make a pound of saffron! Saffron was introduced to Spain from Persia by the Arabs, and thence its use in cooking passed to Europe. It was known to both the Greeks and the Romans, however, and it said to have been the *karcom* mentioned in the Song of Solomon.

Saffron should be used in extremely small quantities in cooking, for a little goes a very long way. The general amount is from ¼ to ½ teaspoon per dish. It may be added to fish and seafood stews, chicken stews, pilafs, and savory rice dishes, and is a must in risotto and paella.

Risotto Milanese

2 tablespoons butter	4 to 5 cups hot chicken or beef stock
1 small onion, finely chopped	Fried chicken livers
1 cup raw rice	½ cup grated Parmesan cheese
1 small pinch saffron	

Melt the butter in a saucepan, and fry the onion in it to a golden brown. Add the rice and stir until it has absorbed the butter. Then add the saffron to the stock, and pour the stock slowly into the rice over a 15-minute period, stirring continuously, until the rice has absorbed all the liquid. Place the rice in a serving dish and top it with the chicken livers and Parmesan cheese.

SAGE

Sage is used chiefly for seasoning fatty meats (pork, goose, duck, sausage), but it can also be used to rub on any beef, lamb, or veal before roasting. It is a good herb to add to marinades, too. Chicken dredged in a mixture of 1 teaspoon sage to 1 cup flour and deep-fried is delicious. Any seafood chowders or chicken soups take sage well, as do a number of vegetables: eggplant, lima beans, onions, peas, potatoes, squash, and tomatoes. Toss them with a pinch of sage mixed with a tablespoon of butter just before serving. Cream cheeses taste particularly good if a little fresh sage is chopped into them (ideally with a silver knife) before serving. Sage has a fairly overpowering taste, hence its use on rich, oily foods. It does a curious and tasty thing, however, when combined with spearmint in pork recipes, for the mint in some miraculous way seems to cancel out the sage's more pungent overtones. It is a difficult thing to describe. Try it and you will see what I mean:

Marian Barnett's Braised Pork

This is an ideal recipe for those confronted by a pork roast, a stove with no oven, and their own sage and spearmint plants. (Dried herbs can be used, but they are not so good.) It also happens to be one of the most delicious and easy ways of preparing pork I have encountered.

1 pork roast (any cut)	1 sprig mint
1 tablespoon bacon fat	2 to 4 cloves garlic, peeled
1 tablespoon olive oil	Salt and freshly ground
2 tablespoons water	black pepper to taste
30 fresh sage leaves	

Brown the pork roast well on all sides in a deep pan over a high flame, using the bacon fat. Lower the heat, pour off all the fat, and add the olive oil, water, sage and mint leaves, whole garlic cloves, salt, and pepper. Cover tightly and cook on the lowest heat for three hours, or until the pork is tender. Serve with rice or mashed potatoes plus a green vegetable. It's fabulous.

Old-fashioned Sage and Onion Sauce, c. 1821

For serving with roast pork, goose, duck, or green peas:

1 tablespoon finely chopped fresh sage, or 1 large pinch dried
2 tablespoons finely chopped onion
4 tablespoons water
Salt and freshly ground black pepper to taste
2 tablespoons bread crumbs
½ cup chicken or beef stock

Simmer the sage and onions in the water for 10 minutes, then add the salt, pepper, and bread crumbs. Stir well, and add the stock. Bring to a boil and simmer for 3 minutes longer before serving.

SAVORY

Summer and winter savory leaves taste identical for all practical purposes, although many cooks like to reserve the tougher and more aromatic winter variety for long-cooking stews and meatloaves, using the summer for vegetables and soups. Savory may be added to any egg dish or omelet, any chicken dish, and rubbed on the surface of any roast meat prior to cooking. When employed in meat stews or soups, again of any variety, add the herb 10 minutes before the cooking time has elapsed. Tomato, potato, and green salads taste excellent with a little freshly chopped savory as a garnish, and any type of gravy or stuffing takes it well. Its most famous and time-honored use is to flavor beans, peas, or lentils, hence its other names *Bohnenkraut* or beanherb. Similarily, a little savory in butter can be used to season cauliflower, eggplant, squash, cabbage, and turnips before serving. In the past it was used as a seasoning for trout, and indeed it can be used with good results on any baked or broiled fish, or in any seafood chowder or casserole. One fourth teaspoon of the dried herb is usually enough for 4 servings.

Lima Beans with Savory

Remove the outer husks of the lima beans, and boil rapidly in salted water until tender—about 20 minutes. Toss them in butter and a large pinch of savory before serving.

Savory Trout

4 to 6 trout	1 large pinch of dried savory,
Milk	or 1 teaspoon chopped fresh
½ teaspoon salt	½ cup flour
1 large pinch ground black pepper	Cooking oil
	⅔ cup butter

Clean and prepare trout, removing the fins (and the heads and tails if you're squeamish). Dip them in milk and dredge them in a mixture of the salt, pepper, savory, and flour. Fry the fish in the cooking oil and brown them well on both sides, and set on a heated serving dish. Discard the oil, but add the butter to the pan now and mix it in with the frying residue over a low heat. Cook until golden brown, and pour over the trout. Serve with parsley sprigs and lemon wedges as garnish.

Savory Stuffing Herbs

For use in any poultry stuffings, mix equal parts marjoram and savory with half parts basil, thyme and tarragon.

SESAME SEEDS

Sesame seeds should be toasted before using in exactly the same manner as poppy seeds (q.v.). They have a similar nutty flavor and may be used in a comparable way on breads, rolls, and cookies; in cheese spreads or to roll soft cheeses in; over salads, or to top casseroles instead of bread crumbs. They and a little butter may be used with good effect to toss green beans, carrots, boiled potatoes, and squash in before serving (1 to 2 teaspoons = 4 servings). Try sprinkling them on spinach as a variation. Chicken and duck coated with 2 tablespoons sesame seeds before roasting is an old Chinese favorite. According to Richard Lucas, the well-known author of books on herbs, sesame seeds are rich in certain sexually stimulating minerals. Whether or not this turns out to be the case, they certainly have been valued extremely highly in the Near East for countless centuries, and it is tempting to believe it was not only for their taste and the oil that was extracted from them.

Be that as it may, whether these cookies turn you on or not, they certainly taste good with ice cream:

Sesame Cookies

2 cups sifted flour	½ cup softened butter
¼ teaspoon nutmeg	1 egg
1 teaspoon baking powder	2 tablespoons toasted
¼ teaspoon salt	sesame seeds
¾ cup granulated sugar	2 tablespoons water

Sift the flour, nutmeg, baking powder, and salt together. Cream the sugar and butter with the egg and add the sesame seeds. Mix in with the flour and water. Chill the dough in the refrigerator for 3 hours, and drop onto an ungreased cookie sheet. Bake in a 375° F. oven until lightly browned—about 10 minutes.

SPEARMINT

Spearmint is used chiefly to flavor cordials, juleps, and jellies. However, it also makes a delicious seasoning for fresh peas or boiled new potatoes. Simply throw a sprig of fresh spearmint into the vegetables 10 minutes before they finish cooking. Roast lamb with mint sauce or mint jelly is a fine old English delicacy. Fresh spearmint leaves may also be used in green salads to give them a different and intriguing flavor.

Mint Sauce

3 sprigs fresh spearmint
1 cup malt or red wine vinegar
1 teaspoon sugar
¼ teaspoon salt

Chop the spearmint leaves finely. Mix the vinegar, sugar, and salt, bring it to a boil in a pan, and pour over the mint leaves. Let the sauce steep for several days before using it with lamb as a table condiment.

Mint Jelly

Also used as a lamb condiment, mint jelly is very simply made by simmering 2 tablespoons finely chopped spearmint in 1 cup redcurrant or apple jelly.

Mint Pasties

An unusual and tasty Yorkshire dessert or teatime pasty can be composed with spearmint in the following manner:

4 cups sifted flour	Grated rind of 1 lemon
4 tablespoons white sugar	1 cup chopped spearmint
1 pinch salt	1 cup currants
4 egg yolks	1 cup brown sugar
2 cups butter	

Sift the flour, white sugar and salt together, and loosely work in the egg yolks, butter, and lemon rind. Add enough water to roll the dough into a ball. Chill for at least 1 hour in the refrigerator; roll out in 2 sheets, filling 6 tart shells with one, reserving the other for the tart coverings. Mix the spearmint with the currants and the brown sugar, and fill each tart with it. Cover with the remaining pastry, pressing the lower and upper crusts together with a fork, and bake in a preheated 450° F. oven until golden brown—about 15 minutes.

TARRAGON (*Artemisia dracunculus*)

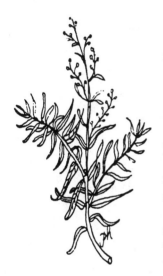

Tarragon is one of the most exclusive and important herbs in French haute cuisine. Its taste is so special that its leaves are frequently used alone and unadulterated by any other herb or spice. It works a particular magic with any chicken, game, or savory omelet, although it can also be used on baked or broiled fish, lamb, and pork chops, in any marinade, on duck, and in any white sauce or mayonnaise! Seafood, tomato, mushroom, consommé, and chicken soups all benefit from the addition of a pinch or two of tarragon 10 minutes before cooking time has elapsed.

Tartar Sauce

A classic and delicious accompaniment to any fried fish:

1 cup real mayonnaise
1 tablespoon chopped shallots
  or chives
1 tablespoon chopped fresh parsley
1 teaspoon finely chopped tarragon

1 tablespoon capers
1 small sweet pickle, finely chopped
1 hard-boiled egg, finely chopped
1 dash lemon juice
1 clove garlic, finely chopped

Combine all the ingredients and blend well. Makes about 1⅓ cups.

Tarragon Eggs Florentine

A tempting appetizer for any dinner menu:

> Previously cooked chopped and buttered spinach
> Butter
> Tarragon
> Salt and freshly ground black pepper
> Eggs at room temperature

Preheat oven to 350° F. Butter 1 individual ramekin or small fireproof soufflé dish for each person, and line it with spinach. Break 1 egg in each dish on top of the spinach, and season with salt, pepper, and a pinch of tarragon (ideally freshly chopped, but dried will do). Bake until the egg whites have whitened—10 to 15 minutes—and serve immediately.

Chicken and Tarragon

> 1 cut-up frying chicken
> Salt and freshly ground black pepper to taste
> ¼ cup flour
> ¼ cup butter
> 1 tablespoon chopped shallots or scallions
> ¼ cup white wine
> 1 teaspoon freshly chopped tarragon, or ½ teaspoon dried
> ¼ cup chicken stock
> ¼ cup heavy cream

Dredge the chicken pieces in salt, pepper, and flour, and fry them in a pan containing ¼ cup of butter until brown on all sides. Transfer them to a heated dish, and fry the shallots lightly in the pan. Then add the wine and stir the sauce briskly over a high flame until most of the liquid has evaporated, making sure to incorporate all the scraps of flour and particles left behind from the chicken. Stir in the remaining dredging flour and the tarragon and slowly add the stock. Now return the chicken to the pan, cover tightly, and allow it to simmer until the chicken is tender—about 40 minutes. Just prior to serving, transfer the chicken to the serving dish and stir the heavy cream into the sauce. Bring it back to a boil, and pour over the chicken. Serve with rice, noodles, or potatoes and green vegetables.

THYME

There are, as we have already seen, an almost endless variety of different-flavored thymes. For now we shall concentrate on the brand usually sold in groceries: regular common or garden thyme. Although a most versatile herb, its field of activity is limited to savory dishes. It can be, and is, used in practically everything. All vegetable juices, egg dishes, cream cheeses, meats, poultry, salads, baked fish, seafoods, and nearly all soups take thyme well. Most green vegetables go well with it, as do carrots, tomatoes, onions, and eggplant. Sausage meats and stuffings are frequently seasoned with thyme. It is an herb no cook should be without.

Baked Veal Chops with Thyme

½ cup sliced onions
½ cup finely chopped carrots
1 large pinch dried thyme, or 1 teaspoon fresh
Loin veal chops
Chicken stock
Salt and freshly ground black pepper to taste
Flour

Preheat the oven to 375° F. Make a bed of vegetables and thyme on the bottom of an ovenproof dish and place the veal chops on top of it. Barely cover with stock, and add salt and pepper. Bake until the chops are brown and tender (about 1¼ hours), turning and basting every ½ hour. Thicken the gravy in the dish with a little flour or cornstarch before serving.

Savory Cream Cheese

1 teaspoon fresh thyme
1 teaspoon fresh chives
1 teaspoon fresh sage
1 clove garlic, crushed
Cream cheese

Chop the herbs finely with a silver knife and incorporate them well with the crushed garlic into the cream cheese. Serve with crackers as an hors d'oeuvre or to round the meal off.

VANILLA

Vanilla is, I suppose, probably the most delicious spice of all. It is certainly one of the most popular. Its use is, however, limited entirely to sweet dishes and desserts. The bean from which the cooking extract is derived is fermented and cured for 6 months before it appears in shops, and the extract itself is prepared by steeping the bean in an alcohol solution to draw out the essential oil. It should only be added to food after cooking, as the flavor is very fugitive and disappears when heated. Curiously enough, unlike many other herbs and spices, the taste of vanilla extract improves with age. A good old Viennese formula to remember when flavoring desserts is: 2 parts vanilla extract to 1 part almond extract. Try flavoring your coffee with a small piece of vanilla bean too, and see how delicious it becomes. Powdered vanilla bean or vanilla extract can be added to any sweet sauce, cooked fruit, compote, or ice cream. Incidentally, you can make your own superior brand of vanilla extract by steeping vanilla beans in cooking brandy.

White Vanilla Sauce

For use over any fruit or pudding:

¼ cup white sugar
1 tablespoon cornstarch
1 cup water

1 inch vanilla bean,
  or 2 teaspoons extract
2 tablespoons butter

Combine the sugar, cornstarch, and water in a double boiler and stir them till they begin to thicken. Remove from the heat and stir in the vanilla and butter. Makes about 1 cup.

Vanilla Cream Pastry Filling

1 tablespoon flour
1 tablespoon sugar
1 egg yolk
½ cup cream
1 teaspoon vanilla extract

Blend the flour, sugar, egg yolks, and cream in a double boiler, stirring continuously. Remove from the heat when thickened, and add the vanilla.

Eating Adventurously

There still remains a large selection of herbs once employed in cooking most of which have since dropped out of general English and American usage. A lot of them, however, are still employed in European Continental cookery, and in certain exotic non-European dishes. Many of them are what one might call acquired tastes, but if you enjoy experimenting with herbs and pride yourself on your inventiveness, you should try them. Also included are a list of the rarer spices with their uses. Again, if you are an adventurous cook, and see them in a store or on a mail-order list, you can do no harm by trying them at least once.

Angelica

Angelica seeds may be used in pastry in the same way as those of anise. Or, if you grow the herb itself, it may be made into an unusual preserve, or candied for inclusion in Christmas cookies.

Angelica Preserve

Cut the trimmed angelica stems into 6-inch-long strips and steep them in boiling water until they soften. Transfer them to cold water and soak for an additional 12 hours. Place 1½ pounds white sugar to every 2 pounds angelica in a pan, separately, and add enough water just to cover it. Bring it to a boil, and add the drained angelica. Continue to boil, testing repeatedly to find the point at which the angelica begins to gel. Bottle and store.

Candied Angelica

This is a somewhat protracted process, but will appeal to those who enjoy pottering in the kitchen. Cut the angelica stalks into 6- to 8-inch chunks. Plunge them in boiling water until they soften, then cool under cold water, drain, and peel off the stringy, celerylike outer fibers. Now soak them in 1 cup white sugar mixed with 1 cup water (more if needed) for 24 hours, at which point drain the liquid off and boil it separately in a pan. When it reaches the temperature of 225° F., pour it over the angelica again. Repeat this process of straining and boiling for three consecutive days. On the fourth, bring the syrup to 245° F., add the angelica itself to the pan and bring to a vigorous boil. Remove the pan, let it cool and discard the syrup. (It may be very effectively used thinned with water and flavored with lemon and brandy as a delicious cordial.) Lay the now translucent green stems on a cookie sheet, sprinkle them with confectioner's sugar, and dry them in a slow oven before canning for storage and later use.

Apple Mint

Use as a garnish. Also try adding a few chopped leaves to applesauce.

Balm

Float sprigs of fresh balm in any punch, lemonade, or claret cup. Its lemony scent and juicy green leaves will add a delightful summery quality to the drink. (See Herb Cordials, p. 175.)

Bergamot

Try chopping the freshly picked leaves and sprinkling them on fruit compotes. Or float a couple of sprigs in any cold punch or summer lemonade.

Borage

Fresh borage has an interesting cucumberlike flavor. Its leaves can be used in salads or white sauces for fish, and both leaves and attractive blue flowers may be floated on top of punch bowls. The leaves were once boiled and served as a table vegetable that tasted rather like spinach.

Burnet

You may also use the tender center leaves of your burnet herb to flavor salads. Like borage, they have a cucumber flavor. The outer leaves tend to be on the bitter side, so be selective. To make an unusual burnet vinegar, pour 1 quart vinegar over ½ ounce of dried, bruised burnet seeds. Bottle and use after 10 days.

Calamus

Calamus is another name for the root of sweet sedge, flag, or gladdon, an aromatic reedlike aquatic plant that flourishes in and around lakes and damp ditches. The essential oil produced from the root is sweet and spicy, and an ounce of the dried root itself has long been considered to make an excellent digestive tea when infused in a pint of boiling water. The root is also widely employed in Indian cookery as a spice. If you wish to try it, use it like ginger root, either with ginger or in place of it.

Camomile

Try a handful of camomile flowers to season your beef stocks.

Canella

Sometimes referred to as white or wild cinnamon or white wood, canella will give you a flavor resembling a pungent, slightly bitter mixture of clove and cinnamon. It was introduced to Europe from the West Indies by the Spaniards during the early seventeenth century, but is now chiefly used on meat in Caribbean cooking. Try adding a little to pipe tobacco and see how fragrant it makes it.

Capers

Capers are the pickled buds of the *Capparis Spinosa*, a plant cultivated chiefly in France, Italy, and Spain. The smaller the bud, the better the flavor, hence they are generally graded, the best being known as "nonpareils" and "capuchins." Use capers in any of your savory white sauces, especially on lamb or fish. They are an essential ingredient in tartar sauce.

Caraway-scented Thyme

Delicious sprinkled on salads and sandwiches.

Carnation

The sweet scent of clove carnations can, like that of many other fragrant garden flowers, be captured in a syrup and used in cordials or over desserts. The only requirement for this eighteenth-century recipe is an abundance of flowers. Simply wash the freshly gathered carnation heads, remove their husks, stems, and heels, and soak them in 5 pints boiling water to every 3 pounds of flowers for 12 hours. Then, without pressing the flowers, strain off the liquid and dissolve in it 2 pounds white sugar to every pint of liquid. Boil rapidly and reduce to a scented syrup.

Cassia

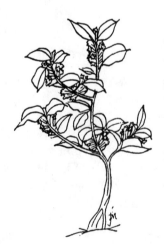

When you buy cinnamon in a store, you can be fairly sure you are buying cassia, *Cinnamomum cassia* a spice from Sumatra, Ceylon, Java, Mexico, or South America. Real cinnamon, *Cinnamomum zeylanicum* comes from Ceylon only, and is very rarely obtainable. However, the smell and taste, for all practical purposes, is identical. Cassia buds may be used to flavor pickles, spiced fruit and in effect anything you would generally put cinnamon in.

Clary Sage

Clary sage possesses an aroma similar to but more perfumed than common sage. You can use it in soups to give them a delicate woodsy flavor. In Germany it is known as muscatel sage: a handful of clary sage leaves and a handful of elder flowers steeped in any Rhenish wine give it a distinct muscatel taste.

Corsican Mint

Use this in iced punches, in fruit salads, with lamb or fish, and as garnish.

Costmary

Tanacetum balsamita, to give costmary its Latin name, is a close relative of the tansy (q.v.). Also known as bible leaf in the United States, it is an aromatic herb with astringent and antiseptic qualities. Nowadays it is chiefly used in sachets and potpourris, although once it was a favorite ingredient of many herbal beers and ales; hence another of its old names, alecost. Its flavor is something like a cross between mint and chrysanthemum. Use it sparingly in soups, broths, or salads.

Cubebs (Cubeba officinalis)

A small spice berry from a Javanese shrub used in perfumery and cooking. Try using it instead of black pepper.

Dandelion

Young dandelion leaves make an interesting bitter addition to any salad. Ideally they should be blanched like chicory. This can be accomplished easily enough by inverting flowerpots over the young plants to exclude any light. Only the whitest and most crisp leaves should be used.

Elderberry and Elder Flower

The flowers, young shoots, and berries of the elder tree may all be used in cookery. A delicious jam and a potent wine can be made from the berries (see Herb Wines, p. 169), while the tender green shoots can be boiled as an effective spinach substitute. Two pounds of the dried flowers steeped in vinegar for 8 days give it an unusual caperlike flavor.

Elderberry Jam

To every pound of berries add ½ cup water, the juice of 2 lemons, and 1 pound white sugar. Boil rapidly until the jam begins to gel, usually between 30 and 40 minutes. (Try mixing this jam with apples. They make a really delicious filling for pies with an authentic country flavor.)

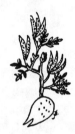

Fenugreek

Fenugreek has a bitter, celerylike flavor. It often appears as a component in curry powders, and is an herb much used in North African and Egyptian cooking. Try using a few crushed seeds in cheese dip.

Filé Powder

If you want to cook Creole style, you'll need filé powder. It is the primary seasoning in all gumbos. To make it mix the dried young leaves of the *Sassafras variifolium*, okra, sage, and coriander, all pounded fine. Thyme and marjoram may also be added, either singly or in combination.

Galangal

Galangal root has been used in Europe as a spice and a perfume for over a thousand years. Its name derives from a Chinese word meaning "mild ginger," and its peppery, gingery taste may be used instead of or in combination with ginger.

Geraniums, Scented (Pelargoniums)

The fresh leaves of scented geraniums (rose, lemon, nutmeg, or apple) may be used to impart fragrance to jellies, jams, punches, or fruit cups. Also try apple-scented geranium leaves in baked apples;

lemon-scented ones in custards. For that matter, lavender flowers, rosemary leaves, verbena, thyme, marjoram, mint, balm, and sage can all be used to flavor any fruit jam or jelly to produce intriguing new flavor combinations.

Grains of Paradise

Sometimes known as Guinea grains or melegueta pepper, these aromatic seeds were once used as an adulterant to black pepper, but are now used only to flavor wine, beer, vinegar, and cordials.

Horehound

White horehound, although generally considered a medicinal herb (q.v.) can also be used to make an old-time confection. The taste is difficult to describe if you've never tried it, but it used to be considered a favorite of country candy stores.

Horehound Candy

Boil the fresh herb down until the juice is extracted, strain, and add an equal amount of white sugar to the remaining liquid. Boil rapidly until the syrup is thick enough to pour into paper molds.

Horseradish

If you like hot, spicy condiments you'll enjoy freshly grated horseradish root as a sauce for cold roast beef, oysters, shrimp, and any oily fish.

Hyssop

Hyssop is a bitter herb with a spicy, minty flavor. If you don't mind a bitter edge to foods, try the freshly chopped young leaves in small quantities on salads and in kidney recipes.

Lemon Grass

This will give a sweet, lemon flavor to any sauces, pickles, and tisanes. The center of the juicier stalks may be used to flavor curries.

Lemon Verbena

Apart from its use as a fragrant medicinal tea, you can use fresh lemon verbena to flavor fruit compotes, punches, and cordials. Try adding the dried leaves to any regular China or Indian tea to give it extra zing.

Lilacs

Lilacs, like violets and roses, may be candied and eaten as a confection (see Roses).

Marigold

The dried petals of marigolds (*Calendula officinalis*) have long been used by herbalists in cooking as well as in medicine. The bright-yellow dye they produce makes them a good substitute for saffron, and they were frequently employed during the seventeenth century to season soups and broths in winter.

Marigold Coffee Cakes

1 teacup milk	4 ounces sugar
1 small handful of	1 small pinch salt
dried marigold petals	3 ounces butter
1 egg	3 ounces lard
1 pound flour	1 handful sultanas
1 teaspoon baking powder	and candied peel

Heat the milk in a pan, and infuse the marigold petals in it while it cools. Strain, discard the petals, and reserve the milk. Beat the egg well, and add it to the milk when it is cool. Mix the flour, baking powder, sugar, and salt well, work in the butter and shortening, and finally add the egg and milk. Mix the sultanas and peel, and blend well, either by hand or better still with an electric blender. Empty into a cake tin, and bake in a moderate oven until the cakes begin to turn a deep golden brown.

Mugwort (Artemisia vulgaris)

Try using a little of this sparingly on pork, duck or goose.

Nasturtium

Flowers, seeds, and petals may be used in place of capers in pickles, soups, and sauces. Chop up a few leaves and sprinkle them on green salads.

Nettles (*Urtica dioica* or *urens*)

The young tops cooked and served with nutmeg and butter make a good substitute for spinach.

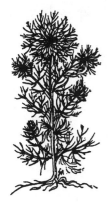

Nigella

Also known as black cumin, and *quatre épices* (four spices) in French cookery, nigella seeds come from the fennel flower, or devil-in-the-bush plant, a member of the Ranunculus (buttercup) family. The pungent, aromatic seeds can be used instead of pepper. *Damascene nigella,* another variety, has seeds which are used in the Near East to sprinkle on top of cakes and breads like sesame.

Orange Mint

Use this dried to spike up any Indian or China tea. Or use a fresh sprig to flavor any jelly or preserve, or float on top of cordials.

Oriental Garlic

Chop the leaves like chives and sprinkle them on baked potatoes and in cheese dips.

Pennyroyal

Try a little of the fresh herb floated on top of cordials. Generally considered a little too pungent for use in cooked food.

Peppermint

Dried peppermint leaves with lemon verbena make a delicious tea to serve hot or cold.

Pineapple Mint

Try chopping a few leaves and sprinkling them on fruit salad.

Pineapple Sage

Add the fresh leaves to any jelly, fruit salad, or cordial.

Pine Nuts

These are used extensively in Italian cooking. They give an exquisite "Roman" taste to any spaghetti sauce. (See basil, above.)

Primrose

Primroses were used in innumerable recipes by cooks in the seventeenth century. The fresh blossoms were frequently made into syrups and tarts, and the young leaves were incorporated into salads as well.

Primrose Syrup

For every 3 pounds fresh flowers, add 5 pints boiling water, then simmer with sugar until a thick syrup is formed. Use it over vanilla ice cream or as an additive to teas.

Purslane

Also known as pussley, the fresh leaves of the common or winter purslane (Portulaca oleracea) may be chopped up and eaten in salads, cooked and served with butter in the manner of French beans, or pickled in vinegar and salt as a garnish. Gerard claimed its use in salads "cools the blood and causes appetite."

Rocket (Hesperis Matronalis)

Once considered a potent aphrodisiac, rocket cress is now used chiefly in Germany and France as a salad garnish. Its taste is strong and sharp. Use only a very small quantity of its fresh leaves. Large doses have a definite emetic effect, and some herbalists utilize it as a substitute for ipecacuanha root.

Roses

Eating roses became a fashionable European pastime during the sixteenth and seventeenth centuries. As a dessert they were considered a great delicacy. Not only were the whole flowers candied, but the petals were turned into jam, honey, wine, and confectionery, and the berries into syrup and tart fillings. Although the demand for the flowers as edibles dwindled, the syrup remained popular until the nineteenth century. Sauce Eglantine, a syrup made from wild rose hips (berries), was one of Queen Victoria's favorite dessert sauces. During the Second World War, when vitamin C was discovered to exist in large quantities in the rose hip, the demand increased considerably. Today rose hip syrup is easily purchasable in most pharmacies. Culpeper was one among many of the early herbalists who recognized the mysterious power of roses to combat infection and hemorrhage, a power we know today to be directly attributable to the presence of from ten to one hundred times as much ascorbic acid in rose hips as there is in most other fruit. "The old conserve," wrote Culpeper, "mixed with 'aromaticum rosarum' [Essence of Roses] . . . is a preservative in time of infection. The dry conserve, which is called the sugar of roses, strengthens the heart and spirits, and stays defluxions [hemorrhages]. The syrup of dried roses . . . comforts the heart, and resists putrefaction and infection, and helps to stay laxes and fluxes."

Roses are in fact, as healthful as they are delicious, the healthful properties being mostly confined to the hip, the delicious ones to the essential oil bearing blossom.

A *Simple Honey of Roses*

Infuse four ounces of dried red rosebuds in one quart of boiling distilled water for six hours. Strain, and mix in five pounds of clarified honey. Boil down to a syrup. Use on bread, toast, desserts or in cookies.

Sauce Eglantine

Wash and scrape the seeds carefully from the insides of 1 cup hips from the wild briar or the dog rose. Purée the hips in a blender, sweeten with ¾ cup sugar (more or less to taste), and add 2 teaspoons lemon juice. Add 1 cup water and bring slowly to a boil, ideally in the top of a double boiler. Separately mix 2 teaspoons cornstarch with 1 tablespoon cold water, and stir this into the hot eglantine sauce. Serve hot or cold over desserts or ice cream.

Rose Candy, or Sugar of Roses [3]

"Take the deepest-coloured red Roses [4] pick them, cut off the white buttons and dry your red leaves [i.e., petals] in an oven, till they be as dry as possible, then beat them to a powder, and searse [sift] them, then take a halfe pound of sugar beaten fine, put it into your pan with as much fair water as will wet it, then set it in a chafing dish of coals and let it boyle till it be sugar again; then put [add] as much powder of the Roses as will make it look very red, stir them well together, and when it is almost cold, put it into pales [open pots] and when it is thoroughly cold, take them off and put them in boxes." (For extra flavor, use rose water instead of "fair water.")

Whole Crystallized Roses

Dissolve 2 ounces powdered gum arabic (obtainable from a pharmacy) in 1 cup water in a double boiler, and let it cool to room temperature. Wash the rose blossoms gently, trimming the stem off close to the base of the bud. Stick a toothpick into each base in place of the stem, and after the blossoms have drained dip each one in the gum arabic solution so that it receives a thorough coating. Allow each to dry for at least 1½ hours; you can stick the toothpick into a styrofoam base or a flower frog to hold them upright.

Mix a few drops of red food coloring into 1 cup white sugar to give it the approximate color of the roses, adding a little yellow or

[3] From *Delights for Ladies*, by Sir Hugh Platt (1594).
[4] Rose petals or buds used in medicine and cookery have to be red or deep pink in color.

purple as the case may be to bring it to a scarlet or carmine tint if necessary. Stir the sugar well to get a thorough color distribution, before spreading it on waxed paper to stand for 30 minutes.

Combine 1 cup water with 2 cups white sugar and 2 tablespoons white corn syrup and bring it to the boil, cooking it until a temperature of 234° F. is reached. Allow to cool, and when lukewarm dip each rose in the mixture, drain it and sprinkle it with the colored sugar. Allow 15 minutes for drying, before removing the toothpick and placing the candied blossoms on the remaining sugar on the paper. Leave for at least 8 hours to complete drying before storing in airtight containers.

Rose Hips

Sprinkle chopped, seeded rose hips on fruit compotes to add a tart flavor, or steep them in wine and use it to deglaze hare or game gravies.

Safflower (Carthamus tinctorius)

Also known as American saffron and fake saffron. Safflower seeds yield a useful cooking oil, while the flowers are used chiefly in dyeing for producing various shades of crimson and scarlet. They can also be used to adulterate real saffron, although many Mexican and Spanish recipes call for safflower as a food coloring. It lacks the fine saffron taste, however, being another genus of plant altogether.

Samphire (Crithmum maritimum)

Otherwise known as sea fennel, sampier, crest marine, and (in Italy) sanpetra, samphire is a succulent green herb that grows close to the sea, often amid stones and rocks. Its strongly aromatic young leaves boiled and covered with vinegar and spice make, according to Mrs. Grieve, one of the very best pickles. Gerard, ever on the lookout for healthful properties, calls samphire pickle a "pleasant sauce for meat, wholesome for the stoppings of the liver, milt and kidnies"!

Sorrel

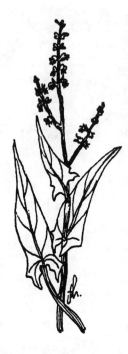

Sorrel leaves are still used extensively in French cookery. As its other names, sourgrass, wood sour, and sour sauce all indicate, fresh sorrel leaves yield an acid taste which adds an interesting overtone to green salads. "Sorrell imparts so grateful a quickness to the salad that it should never be left out," wrote the seventeenth-century herbalist John Evelyn. There are basically two types of sorrell you can use in cooking and medicine (sorrel leaves are refrigerant and diuretic): garden sorrel, *Rumex acetosa,* and French sorrel, *Rumex scutatus.* If you wish to grow your own, sow the seeds in spring in any type of soil, and divide the perennial roots in the fall or the following spring. Apart from their use in salads, sorrel leaves may be used in stocks, as a tenderizing seasoning for roast lamb and veal, in turnips, and as a condiment for roast goose or pork instead of applesauce.

French Sorrel Stock, c. 1884

To make a basic cooking stock, take:

3 tablespoons chopped fresh sorrel leaves
1½ tablespoons chopped fresh lettuce leaves
2 teaspoons chopped fresh chervil leaves
3½ cups water
½ teaspoon salt
1 teaspoon butter

Wash and boil the leaves in the water for 20 minutes. Add the salt and butter enrichment, cook for 5 minutes longer, strain, and reserve for later use.

Star Anise

Yields a sweet, licorice flavor. A must in Chinese and Japanese cooking.

Strawberry Leaves

If you grow a strawberry plant in a strawberry pot which is plentiful in leaves but short in berries, this old turkey recipe will put those leaves to good use for you. (Incidentally, you can also infuse them into a pleasantly scented tonic tea: 1 teaspoon dried leaves to 1 cup boiling water.)

Lammas Turkey

"Gather strawberry leaves on Lammas Eve [eve of August 1], press them in the distillery until the aromatic perfume thereof becomes sensible. [Don't bother, just crush them in your pestle and mortar.] Take a fat turkey and pluck him, and baste him, then enfold him carefully in the strawberry leaves. Then boil him in water from the well [tap water is even better these days] and add rosemary, velvet flower [*Amaranthus oleraceus* or *polygonoides*], lavender, thistles [*Onopordon acanthium* or *Silybum marianum*], stinging nettles [*Urtica*] and other sweet-smelling herbs. [These can advantageously be replaced by tarragon, thyme, marjoram, and savory.] Add also a pinte of canary wine [use a Madeira], and half a pound of butter and one of ginger passed through a sieve. Sieve with plums and stewed raisins and a little salt. Cover him with a silver dish cover." [It is actually delicious if you enjoy sweet sauces on poultry.]

Sweet Cicely (Myrrhis odorata)

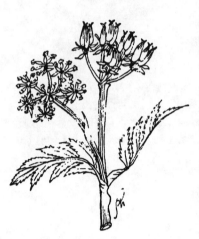

Sweet cicely, sometimes known as sweet chervil, sweet fern, British myrrh, or the Roman plant, is a fragrant perennial herb of the Umbelliferae family. It grows best in moist ground and semishade. Its flavor is sweet and aniselike, and herbalists consider it an excellent sugar substitute in fruit compotes. Its leaves and seeds may be added to diet lemon salad dressings to reduce the tartness, and they go well with raw vegetable juices. Try the seeds in cakes and cookies instead of anise seeds, too. Use 1 teaspoonful of the dry herb to 1 cup liquid or fruit.

Tamarind

Not strictly an herb or spice, but sometimes listed as such, the fruit of the tamarind tree is a native of the West Indies. The pulp from the pods is used in France to prepare a spicy cordial. They should be prepared in the same way as lemonade.

Tansy

Tansy was a popular seasoning herb during the eighteenth century, and was frequently employed in small amounts as a condiment with roast lamb before spearmint took its place. It has a curious bitter flavor, which is probably one of the reasons it was reckoned to be one of the "bitter herbs" eaten by the Jews at Passover. The custom passed into Christian practice with the eating of "tansies," puddings or cakes traditionally eaten during the springtime period of religious abstinence known as Lent. Most "tansies" are savory in character, almost invariably calling for the use of eggs, bread, and spinach juice, and fried like a pancake. None of them are really very appetizing, but then they probably were not meant to be. One old recipe does, however, defy the rule. Far from being a diet of abstinence, it seems rather the reverse:

Tansy Pudding [5]

"Blanch and pound a quarter of a pound of Jordan almonds, put them in a stew pan, add a gill [½ cup] of syrup of Roses [you can use Rose Hip Syrup for this], the crumb of a French roll [i.e., bread crumbs], some grated nutmeg, half a glass of brandy, two tablespoonfulls of tansy juice [you will need the fresh herb for this], three ounces of fresh butter and some slices of citron [lemon]. Pour over it a pint and a half of boiling cream or milk; sweeten and when cold mix it, add the juice of a lemon, and eight eggs beaten. It may be either boyled or baked."

Tonquin Beans

Also known as tonka beans, these large seeds of the *Dipteryx odorata* contain a large proportion of coumarin, the aromatic substance in woodruff so valued by pharmacists and parfumiers. Often used as a substitute or adulterant for vanilla pods, tonka bean may be used to flavor cocoa, ice cream, and candy. Try putting a bean or two in a tobacco can and see how the flavor improves, too.

Trigonella

See Fenugreek.

[5] From *The Good Housewife's Handmaid* (1588).

Turmeric Root (Curcuma longa)

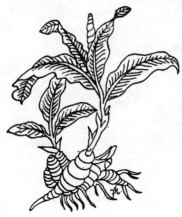

This pungent Indian spice is a close relative of ginger, and an almost indispensable ingredient of genuine curry powder. (See above under Cayenne.) It may also be used to add zap to mayonnaise, sauces, pickles, and mustard. Go easy with it, though, for it is very potent. For medicinal purposes it is recognized as being a stimulant and a digestive.

Violets

Violet flowers may be candied for cake decoration and confectionery, or turned into a syrup or honey. Use the same technique as you would for roses (q.v.), leaving out the toothpick part during crystallization.

Woodruff

Woodruff is used chiefly in sachets and to flavor wines and cordials. For the famous woodruff Maybowl recipe, see p. 179.

Wormwood

A close relative of mugwort (q.v.), used in a similar manner.

Yarrow

A few of the fresh young leaves chopped and sprinkled on a green salad will give it an aromatic and faintly bitter flavor.

Zedoary

See Turmeric

Zubrovka

Zubrovka grass is grown in Russia and Poland, and is used mainly as an exotic flavoring for vodkas. It can, however, be mixed with any alcoholic beverage to lend it a mellow and aromatic flavor.

Quick Reference Guide to Herb and Spice Flavoring

BEVERAGES

CHOCOLATE AND COCOA. Cinnamon. Cloves. Nutmeg. Tonka. Vanilla pods.

COFFEE. Cardamom. Cinnamon. Cloves. Vanilla pods.

LEMONADE. Balm. Bergamot. Borage. The geraniums. Lemon grass. Lemon verbena. The mints. Pineapple sage. Woodruff.

INDIAN OR CHINA TEA. Lemon grass. Lemon verbena. Orange mint. Rose geranium. Spearmint.

BREADS AND CAKES

BREADS AND ROLLS. Caraway seed. Poppy seed. Sesame seed. Paprika. Oregano. Black pepper. Cinnamon. Cardamom seed. Fennel seed. Anise seed. Sweet cicely seed. Nigella.

CAKES AND COOKIES. Cloves. Nutmeg. Cinnamon. Allspice. Caraway seed. Anise seed. Poppy seed. Sesame seed. Cardamom seed. Sweet nigella. Cicely seed. Vanilla. Tonka. Coriander.

FRUIT

APPLE. Cardamom seed. Cloves. Cinnamon. Nutmeg. Fennel. Vanilla.

APRICOT. Cinnamon. Cloves. Hyssop. Vanilla.

CHERRIES. Allspice. Cinnamon. Vanilla. Cloves. Nutmeg.

CURRANTS. Cinnamon. Clove.

PEACH. Cinnamon. Allspice. Nutmeg. Vanilla.

EGGS, CHEESE, AND PASTA

CHEESE, HOT. Basil. Oregano. Caraway seed. Nutmeg. White pepper. Curry powder. Turmeric, Paprika. Garlic. Cayenne.

CREAM CHEESES. Chives. Chervil. Sage. Thyme. Paprika. Cayenne. Garlic. Savory.

EGGS, CREAMED OR DEVILED. Cayenne. Celery seed. Curry powder. Chives. Chervil. Tarragon. Mustard. Savory. Paprika. Garlic.

EGGS, SCRAMBLED OR IN SOUFFLÉS OR OMELETS. Basil. Chives. Chervil. Dill. Parsley. Savory. Garlic. Thyme. Lovage. Tarragon.

PASTA SAUCES. Black pepper. Parsley. Oregano. Cayenne. Thyme. Caraway seed. Basil. Bay. Marjoram. Pine nuts. Garlic.

SAVORY RICE DISHES. Bay. Saffron. Safflower. Turmeric. Cumin. Paprika. Black pepper. Curry powder. Pine nuts. Marigold petals.

CREAM SAUCES. Paprika. White pepper. Cayenne. Tarragon. Lovage. Nutmeg. Nasturtium. Capers. Sorrel. Borage.

CUSTARDS. Nutmeg. Vanilla. Cinnamon.

FISH

SEA BASS. Shallots. Parsley. Black pepper.

STRIPED BASS. Sage. Thyme. Bay. Shallots. Parsley. Black pepper.

BLUEFISH. Tarragon. Thyme. Parsley. Black pepper. Bay.

CARP. Parsley. Black pepper.

CLAMS. Celery seed. Marjoram. Sage. Savory. Oregano. Thyme. Black pepper. Parsley. Basil. Garlic.

COD. Black pepper. Cumin. Thyme. Bay.

CRAB. Black pepper. Chives. Tarragon. Parsley. Dill seeds. Fennel seeds. Chervil. Oregano. Rosemary.

FLOUNDER. Parsley. Rosemary. Bay. Thyme. Black pepper.

HADDOCK. Black pepper. Marjoram. Oregano.

HALIBUT. Parsley. Bay. Thyme. Tarragon. Black pepper.

LOBSTER. Marjoram. Oregano. Thyme. Garlic.

MACKEREL. Thyme. Parsley. Sesame seeds.

OYSTERS. Marjoram. Savory. Mace. Black, white, and cayenne pepper. Horseradish.

PIKE. Black pepper. Parsley. Paprika.

RED SNAPPER. Parsley. Bay. Thyme. Basil.

SALMON. Black pepper. Dill seeds. Bay. Parsley.

SCALLOPS. Parsley. Black pepper. Rosemary.

SHAD. Thyme. Bay. Black pepper.

SHRIMP. Thyme. Spearmint. Black pepper. Garlic. Chives. Bay. Parsley. Mace. Rosemary. Horseradish. Basil. Tarragon. Oregano. Celery seed.

SNAILS. Garlic. Parsley.

SOLE. Parsley. Black pepper. Chives.

SQUID. Thyme. Parsley. Black pepper. Ginger. Dill.

SWORDFISH. Black pepper. Parsley.

TROUT. Bay. Parsley. Thyme. Garlic.

TUNA. Chervil. Fennel. Thyme. Black pepper.

WHITING. Parsley. Black pepper. Mustard.

MEATS

BEEF. Rosemary. Horseradish. Basil. Paprika. Caraway. Dill. Black pepper. Bay. Thyme. Marjoram. Allspice. Parsley. Ginger. Turmeric. Oregano. Garlic. Savory. Chervil. Calamus. Galangal. Borage.

BRAINS. Basil. Thyme. Bay.

HAM. Cloves. Mustard. Black pepper. Cayenne. Marjoram. Parsley. Dill. Sage.

HARE. Black pepper. Thyme. Juniper berries. Marjoram.

KID OR GOAT. Sage. Bay. Thyme.

KIDNEY. Oregano. Basil. Black pepper. Parsley. Celery seed. Mustard. Rosemary. Garlic. Hyssop.

LAMB. Black pepper. Ginger. Sorrel. Cloves. Parsley. Spearmint. Tansy. Thyme. Bay. Juniper. Tarragon. Oregano. Paprika. Caraway. Cardamom. Cayenne. Cinnamon. Cumin. Dill. Rosemary. Coriander. Turmeric. Chervil. Galangal. Lemon balm. Garlic. Marjoram. Calamus.

LIVER. Black pepper. Thyme. Parsley. Marjoram.

PORK. Rosemary. Sage. Cayenne pepper. Black pepper. Thyme. Nutmeg. Bay. Cloves. Calamus. Fennel seeds. Spearmint. Parsley. Oregano. Chives. Caraway. Mustard. Paprika. Ginger. Coriander. Mugwort. Plantain. Dill. Marjoram. Garlic. Wormwood.

RABBIT. Sage.

SAUSAGE. Rosemary. Sage. Thyme. Oregano. Marjoram. Garlic. Bay. Fennel.

SWEETBREADS. Black pepper.

TONGUE. Bay. Black pepper. Tarragon.

TRIPE. Cloves. Bay. Thyme. Black pepper.

OXTAIL. Nutmeg. Black pepper. Parsley.

VEAL. Thyme. Rosemary. Black pepper. Bay. Parsley. Basil. Calamus. Chervil. Nutmeg. Tarragon. Sage. Chives. Celery seed. Sorrel. Galangal. Lemon balm. Oregano. Ginger. Paprika. Marjoram.

VENISON. Parsley. Bay. Thyme. Juniper. Basil. Black pepper. Coriander. Savory. Celery seed.

POULTRY AND WILDFOWL

CHICKEN. Sesame seed. Tarragon. Garlic. Bay. Cayenne. Paprika. Black pepper. Parsley. Oregano. Galangal. Rosemary. Cumin Thyme. Sage. Marjoram. Calamus. Basil. Celery seed. Savory.

DOVE. Black pepper. Parsley.

DUCK. Black pepper. Thyme. Parsley. Bay. Cinnamon. Sesame seed. Calamus. Anise. Garlic. Ginger. Wormwood. Mugwort.

GOOSE. Black pepper. Wormwood. Mugwort. Rosemary. Bay. Parsley. Caraway seed. Oregano. Sage. Thyme. Savory. Garlic.

GROUSE. Black pepper. Thyme. Bay. Parsley.

PARTRIDGE. Black pepper. Thyme. Bay. Parsley. Garlic.

PHEASANT. Black pepper. Thyme. Tarragon. Savory. Marjoram. Bay. Allspice. Oregano.

PIGEON (SQUAB). Black pepper. Parsley. Bay. Thyme. Garlic.

QUAIL. Same as partridge.

ROCK CORNISH GAME HEN. Same as chicken.

STUFFING. Marjoram. Lemon balm. Thyme. Tarragon. Parsley. Garlic. Celery seed. Savory.

TURKEY. Sesame seed. Paprika. Celery seed. Sage. Black pepper. Mace. Marjoram. Savory. Tarragon. Thyme.

SALAD DRESSINGS

GREEN SALADS. Garlic. Dandelion. Sorrel. Costmary. Yarrow. Spearmint. Tarragon. Rocket. Burnet. Dill. Basil. Lemon balm. Marjoram. Chervil. Purslane. Lovage. Sweet cicely. Borage. Hyssop.

TOMATO SALADS. Basil. Oregano. Garlic. Sweet cicely. Lemon balm. Chervil. Lovage. Borage.

VEGETABLES

ARTICHOKES. Garlic. Dill. Mustard. Bay. Thyme. Parsley. Black pepper. Pine nuts. Oregano.

ASPARAGUS. Black pepper. Thyme. Bay. Basil. Caraway seed. Tarragon.

AVOCADO. Dill weed.

BEANS, GREEN, FRENCH, OR SNAP. Rosemary. Basil. Oregano. Savory. Dill. Parsley. Black pepper.

BROAD. Savory. Dill. Black pepper.

LIMA, FLAGEOLET. Black pepper. Savory. Dill.

HARICOT. Parsley. Black pepper. Cumin. Paprika.

BEETS. Parsley. Black pepper. Horseradish. Basil. Caraway seed. Dill seed. Chervil. Cloves. Thyme.

BROCCOLI. Black pepper. Basil. Caraway seeds. Parsley. Dill seed. Oregano.

BRUSSELS SPROUTS. Dill. Parsley. Black pepper. Caraway seed. Thyme. Marjoram. Cumin. Tarragon. Chives.

CABBAGE. Same as brussels sprouts.

CARROTS. Black pepper. Parsley. Cloves. Nutmeg. Chervil. Caraway seed. Chives. Dill. Spearmint. Basil. Fennel seed. Thyme.

CAULIFLOWER. Dill seed. Mace. Paprika. Parsley. Tarragon. Marjoram.

CELERY. Basil. Black pepper. Parsley. Thyme. Tarragon. Oregano. Chives. Chervil.

CHICORY. Chervil.

CORN. Black pepper.

CUCUMBER. Black and white pepper. Dill. Chervil. Chives. Parsley. Basil. Borage. Thyme. Tarragon.

EGGPLANT. Nutmeg. Paprika. Black pepper. Rosemary. Marjoram.

ENDIVE. Chervil.

ESCAROLE. Black pepper. Pine nuts.

KALE. White pepper.

LEEKS. Parsley. Dill. Celery seed. Black pepper. Bay. Thyme.

LENTILS. Black pepper. Dill. Oregano.

MUSHROOMS. Parsley. Black pepper. Caraway seed. Marjoram. Chives. Coriander seed.

ONIONS. See Leeks.

PEAS. Spearmint. Dill. Black pepper. Chives. Basil. Marjoram. Oregano. Rosemary.

PEPPERS, GREEN. Oregano. Black pepper. Parsley. Marjoram.

POTATOES. Rosemary. Caraway. Spearmint. Black pepper. Nutmeg. Dill. Chives. Paprika. Parsley. Chervil. Basil.

PUMPKIN. Cinnamon.

RUTABAGA (SWEDE). Parsley. Nutmeg. Black pepper. Ginger. Mace.

SPINACH. Oregano. Nutmeg. Black pepper. Sesame seed. Sage. Thyme. Rosemary. Marjoram. Chives.

SQUASH, ACORN. Ginger. Nutmeg. Caraway seed. Black pepper. Mace. Cloves.

SUMMER. Garlic. Oregano. Basil. Caraway seed. Parsley. Black pepper. Fennel seed. Marjoram. Thyme. Pine nuts. Chives.

ZUCCHINI. Tarragon. Parsley. Oregano. Black pepper.

SWEET POTATOES. Cloves. Nutmeg. Cinnamon. Black pepper.

TOMATOES. Basil. Oregano. Black pepper. Bay. Parsley. Chervil. Chives. Dill seed. Thyme. Tarragon.

TURNIPS. Allspice. Parsley. Celery seed. Basil. Paprika. Dill seed. Chives. Caraway seed.

VINEGARS

Any of the following herbs may be steeped in vinegar to give it a flavor. Mix the vinegar with a little oil, salt, and mustard, and use it on any salad.

Samphire. Tarragon. Burnet. Dill. Basil. Spearmint. Lemon balm. Marjoram. Garlic. Chives. Thyme. Savory. Celery seed. Chervil. Fennel. Clary sage. Elder flowers. Nasturtium. Purslane. Sweet cicely.

Herbal Beverages

Herbs and spices were once used extensively in the composition and flavoring of various types of drinks, both alcoholic and nonalcoholic. Old herbals are frequently littered with recipes for these beverages. Some of the old favorites sound pretty disgusting by today's standards: nettle beer, burdock ale, parsnip wine. However, when you think about it, mashed distilled rye, which is all that vodka is, doesn't sound very appetizing either. Obviously it is the end product rather than the process that counts. However, the prospect of being faced with a bubbling hellbroth of squashed nettles, oak leaves, or parsnips is not exactly a tempting one to the beginner, even though you are assured the outcome will prove potent and delicious. I have therefore tried to pick a selection of beverages that sound as well as taste good.

HERB BEERS

Old English and European country inns always used to brew their own beers. Many farmhouses did likewise. Although hops and malt form the basis for beers and ales today, this was not always the case. Practically any herb tea could be fermented and turned into an alcoholic drink. Some taste better than others, however, and these are the ones which have become today's traditional country herb beers and wines. "Beer," "ale," and "wine" are interchangeable words in the area of herbal beverages. Strictly speaking, beer and ale are brewed from fermented malt and hops, wine from grapes. Not so with herbs.

Many herb beers and wines turn out moderately nonalcoholic; others quite the opposite. I can recall particularly potent batches of elderberry wine and ginger beer, drinks often (and quite erroneously) considered mild by the uninitiated. Exactly how your brew will turn out is bound to be a hit-or-miss matter to begin with, depending on the strength of your herbs, how much, if any, yeast you introduce, and the temperature and length of time you allow for fermentation. However, whether your home brew knocks you flat or merely provides mild "uplift," the pride you'll feel in having created an even comparatively tasty and alcoholic beverage of your very own has to be experienced to be believed.

All these recipes are extremely simple. All they require are one or two large enamel kettles (depending on the size you can muster); a wooden tub, large ceramic or enamel basin, or even an old enamel sitz bath, but ideally a small winemaker's cask in which to ferment the liquor, a cloth with which to cover it if you use a basin, and a place to store it. (Never make wines or beers in untreated metal containers, always enamel.) Plus, of course, one or two bottles—old wine bottles will do fine—in which to draw the liquid off after fermentation has ceased.

Agrimony Ale

Take equal amounts of dried dandelion, meadowsweet herb, and agrimony herb. For every ounce of herbs add a gallon of water. Boil for 20 minutes, then strain and add 1 pound sugar per gallon to the liquid. Pour it into a cask or tub (or their equivalent) and float a small piece of toast spread on both sides with 1 cup brewer's yeast. Cover with a cloth or towel and leave to stand in a warm place for 12 hours before drawing off the liquid and bottling.

Camomile Beer

12 ounces camomile	2 ounces burned sugar
4 ounces ground ginger root	4 ounces cream of tartar
5 gallons boiling water	5 gallons cold water
2½ pounds sugar	¼ cup brewer's yeast,
35 grains (just over ½ teaspoon)	spread on both sides of a
saccharine 550	piece of toast

Infuse the camomile and ginger in 5 gallons boiling water in a covered vessel for 15 minutes. Strain; add the plain sugar and saccharine, stirring well, and then the burned sugar, cream of tartar, and 5 gallons cold water. Mix well, and float the toast on the surface of the liquid. Cover and allow to stand between 65° to 70° F. for 12 hours. Then remove the toast and bottle the beer for future use.

Old-fashioned Ginger Beer

A very easy, popular, and rather alcoholic recipe:

5 pounds white sugar
3 ounces ground ginger root
3 gallons water
5 lemons
¼ cup brewer's yeast

Boil the sugar, ginger, and water for 1 hour. Cool, and add the juice and thinly sliced rinds of the lemons. Pour into a tub, and float the yeast spread on both sides of a piece of toast on the surface.

Cover with a thick cloth, and leave to ferment for 2 to 3 days. Strain through cheesecloth or a fine mesh, and bottle, securing the corks tightly by tying them down. Allow at least 5 days before drinking. If you need more bite to it, increase the amount of ginger.

Confederate Ale

4 gallons water
8 ounces molasses
⅛ ounce ground ginger root
1 bay leaf
brewer's yeast, spread on both sides
    of a piece of toast

Boil the first 4 ingredients together for 15 minutes, then cool and tub, floating the yeast-covered toast on the liquid's surface to start the fermentation. Cover with a cloth.

Spruce Beer

½ ounce black spruce
  (*Abies nigra*) twigs
Water
½ ounce ginger root
1 ounce hop flowers

1 ounce sassafras chips
¼ ounce ground allspice
3½ pounds brown sugar
2 cups brewer's yeast

Boil the spruce twigs in a little water for 30 minutes; strain the juice and reserve. Pour enough boiling water over the ginger root to cover, and allow to steep for 24 hours; strain and reserve. Combine the spruce and ginger essences with the hops, sassafras, allspice, and sugar in 5 gallons water and boil for 30 minutes. Tub and cool, then add the yeast. Leave for 24 hours before bottling.

Hop Beer

Even simpler to put together is the following old country standby:

1 ounce hops
½ ounce bruised fresh ginger root
3 pints water
1½ pounds Demerara sugar

Boil the hops and the ginger together in the water for ½ hour. Add the sugar, and continue boiling until it has dissolved. Pour into an open ceramic vessel and let stand overnight. Draw off gently and bottle. Should be drunk before 1 week.

Horehound Beer

6 ounces horehound
2 pounds treacle
3 gallons water
2 tablespoons brewer's yeast,
    spread on both sides of a piece of toast

Boil the first 3 ingredients together for 1 hour, strain, and cool to lukewarm. Float the brewer's yeast spread on toast on the surface, and let stand for 24 hours before bottling.

Meadowsweet Ale

This old beverage, more in the nature of a cordial than a beer, makes use of the long recognized virtues of meadowsweet, a fragrant herb valued in home brewing since the sixteenth century.

2 ounces meadowsweet	3 gallons water
2 ounces agrimony	2½ pounds white sugar
2 ounces betony	½ ounce hyssop
2 ounces raspberry leaves	

Boil all the herbs save the hyssop in the water for 15 minutes. Strain, add the sugar and hyssop, and mix well. When cool, strain once more and bottle. No yeast need be added.

Three Flowers Beer

An old French country drink may be made out of hops, violets, and elder blossoms:

1 ounce hops flowers	4½ pounds brown sugar
1 ounce violet flowers	1 cup white wine vinegar
1 ounce elder flowers	¼ ounce brewer's yeast,
11 quarts water	spread on both sides of a piece of toast

Boil the flowers in 11 quarts water for 5 minutes, and then strain. Add the sugar and vinegar and mix well. Pour into a tub or barrel and float the toast in it. Leave for 2 days to ferment before drawing off the liquid and bottling for future use.

HERB WINES

Herb wines are a little more sophisticated than beers, but really just as easy to make. Whereas most beers and ales take no more than a week, or two at most, to ferment, wines need anything from 3 months to a year or two to produce a good vintage.

Balm Wine

10 pounds white sugar
4 gallons water
1¼ pounds fresh balm tops
2 tablespoons brewer's yeast
Sugar lumps

Boil the sugar in the water for 1¼ hours, skimming carefully. Bruise the balm tops and place them in a small cask or tub with 2 tablespoons brewer's yeast. When the sugar water has cooled, pour it over the balm, stirring the mixture well. Let stand for 24 hours, stirring every 4 hours or so. Cover the cask lightly until the fermentation ceases—about 9 weeks—and draw off the liquid into bottles, placing a lump of sugar in each bottle. Cork firmly, and store for at least 1 year before using.

Coltsfoot Wine

2 quarts dried coltsfoot flowers
1 gallon water
3 pounds white sugar
3 oranges, sliced
2 lemons, sliced
¼ cup raisins
2 tablespoons brewer's yeast, spread on both sides of a piece of toast

Infuse the coltsfoot flowers in the boiling water, and let them stand for 3 days, stirring 3 times a day. Strain off the liquid at the end of this time, add the sugar, and boil for 30 minutes. Cool and add the yeast spread on toast. Remove the toast the following day and cask, adding the oranges, lemons, and raisins. Let stand for 3 months before bottling.

Dandelion Wine

4 quarts fresh dandelion flowers	Rind of 1 orange
1 gallon cold water	1 lemon, sliced
3½ pounds white sugar	2 tablespoons brewer's yeast, spread
1 piece ginger root	on both sides of a piece of toast

Make sure the dandelion flowers are free of all portions of stem. Place them in a tub and pour 1 gallon *cold* water on them, leaving them to stand for 3 days, stirring every 8 hours or so. Strain off the golden liquid at the end of this time, and boil it with the sugar, ginger, orange, and lemon for 30 minutes. After it has cooled, float the toast on it, cover with a cloth, and leave for 2 days to start the fermentation. Cask with the bung only lightly in place for a week or two until the gases have escaped, and then bung tightly for 2 months before bottling. The wine tastes like a mild sherry.

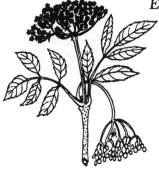

ELDER (*Sambucus niger*)

Elderberry Wine

Vying in popularity with dandelion wine is this old country beverage. Elderberry wine is a delicious spicy drink, rather like a rich port wine. It can be drunk cold in spring and summer or mulled on cold winter days. Ideally elderberries should be gathered on a warm day while the sun is on them, or so many of the old recipes stipulate. This seems to bring out their best flavor.

1 gallon elderberries
2 gallons water
Up to 9 pounds sugar
1½ ounces ginger root
1½ ounces crushed allspice

¾ ounce cloves
2 tablespoons brewer's yeast, spread
on both sides of a piece of toast
1½ cups brandy

Boil the elderberries in the water for 30 minutes, then mash them up and strain them through a fine sieve. Discard the husks. For every gallon of liquid mix in 3 pounds sugar. Put the spices in a small cheesecloth bouquet, and suspend them in the liquid while you bring it to a brisk boil for another 15 minutes. Pour into a basin or tub, discarding the spices, and float the toast on the surface when it has cooled. Cover with a cloth and leave for 2 days, at the end of which time discard the yeast and add the brandy. Cask or store in a large stone jar. May be drunk after 8 weeks, and will last for as long as 8 years if bottled.

Elder Flower Wine

Otherwise known as Frontiniac wine, this recipe dates from the eighteenth century. The original text requires large amounts of ingredients, which I have cut down proportionally. It also calls for syrup of lemons, which amounts simply to lemon juice preserved with sugar. Plain lemon rinds and juice will provide the flavor just as effectively.

3 pounds chopped raisins
6 pounds sugar
3 gallons water

2 quarts fresh elder flowers
Rind and juice of 2 lemons
2 tablespoons brewer's yeast

Boil the raisins and the sugar in the water for 1 hour. Skim, and allow to cool in a tub or basin. When lukewarm, add the elder flowers. Leave for 24 hours before incorporating the lemon rinds and juice. Mix well and add the yeast whole, then cover and let stand for two months before bottling.

English Sack [6]

If I had a thousand sons, the first human
principle I would teach them should be,
to forswear thin potations and to addict
themselves to sack.

[6] Adapted from *The Compleat Housewife,* by E. Smith (1736).

So said Shakespeare's Sir John Falstaff of "sack," or saragossa wine, a name that later came to be applied to any Spanish or Canary white wine or sherry. However, the English had their own "sack" too, and it was made not from grapes but from herbs. Like all really old recipes, it calls for honey as a sweetener instead of sugar.

> 4 sprigs rue
> 1 handful fennel root
> 1 gallon water
> 3 pounds honey

Boil the rue and fennel in the water for 30 minutes, strain, and add the honey. Boil for a further 2 hours, skimming from time to time, before emptying the liquid into a cask. Allow the sack to ferment for 1 year before drawing off and bottling.

Marigold Wine

Here's one good way to use up all the petals from your marigold flowers:

8 pounds sugar	1½ pounds seedless raisins, chopped
2 pounds honey	5 tablespoons brewer's yeast,
3 gallons water	spread on both sides of a piece
Shells and whites of 3 eggs	of toast
8 quarts marigold	1 pint brandy
(*Calendula officinalis*) petals	½ ounce isinglass solution

Boil 7 pounds of the sugar, honey, and water together, and add the shells and whites of the eggs (this is an old culinary secret for clearing any type of liquid or consommé of solid matter). Filter the shells and impurities out through fine muslin, and pour the boiling liquid over the petals and raisins in a tub. Cover it tightly, and leave for 24 hours, at which point stir, re-cover, and let stand for a further 3 days. Place the thinly pared rinds (no white) of 3 oranges and 1 pound white sugar in the bottom of a cask and pour the strained liquid on top. Float the toast on the surface to start the fermentation, and cover the bunghole lightly. When the wine has ceased frothing remove the toast and add 1 pint brandy and ½ ounce isinglass solution, bung the cask firmly, and leave to mature for 3 to 5 months before bottling.

Mead

This is a beverage dating back to the time of the Vikings. Any number of different herbs and spices have been used to brew it, depending on the taste of the brewer. If you don't mind waiting 9 months or so for fermentation to occur, like most herb beers and ales it's really very easy to make. Here is the basic recipe, followed by a list of extra traditional ingredients you can incorporate if you wish.

Whites of 2 eggs	A little bruised ginger
6 quarts water	2 cloves
2½ pounds honey	brewer's yeast, spread on
1 blade mace	both sides of a piece of toast
½ teaspoon powdered cinnamon	

Optional ingredients: Use 1 ounce dried herbs to every gallon of liquid.

Rosemary leaves	Lemon peel	Angelica
Sweetbriar	Marjoram	Wormwood
(*Rosa rubiginosa*)	Elder flowers	Borage
Buckbean	Germander	Ground ivy
Balm	(*Teucrium*	(*Glechoma*
Yarrow	*scorodonia*)	*hederacea*)
Burnet	Spearmint	Bugloss leaves
Thyme	Broom tops	(*Echium vulgare*)

Beat the egg whites and mix them well with the water. Add all the other ingredients and bring to a boil, stirring continuously. Simmer for 1 hour, and then cool. Strain into a tub or cask, add the yeast-spread toast, and cover loosely. Bung the cask tightly only after the fermentation stops. Bottle after 9 months. For extra spiciness, a small cheesecloth bag of cinnamon, ginger, cloves, and nutmeg may be suspended in the cask or tub while the fermentation is taking place.

Primrose Wine

Also known as cowslip wine, this time-honored drink was often prescribed by herbalists as a fragrant sedative, sleeping potion, and headache cure. Again, it is extremely easy to concoct.

2 gallons water
2½ pounds sugar
2 lemons
1 gallon primrose (*Primula veris*) flowers
1 tablespoon brewer's yeast, spread on both sides
   of a piece of toast
Sugar lumps

Boil the water and the sugar together for 30 minutes, skim, and pour into a tub over the rinds of the 2 lemons. When it is cool, add the strained juice of the lemons and the whole primrose flowers and float the yeast-spread toast on the surface. Cover and let stand for 2 days, stirring every 8 hours. Remove the yeast at the end of this time and cask the liquid. Let stand for a further 4 weeks before drawing off into bottles. Place a lump of sugar in each bottle.

Sage Wine

Here is a simple wine in which you can incorporate several of your garden herbs, such as sage, rosemary, lavender, primrose, or carnation heads.

1 gallon water
6 quarts chopped sage leaves or other herb
6 pounds chopped raisins

Boil the water and pour it onto the sage and raisins. Let it stand for 6 days, stirring 2 or 3 times daily. Strain and press the liquor from the ingredients, then cask it for 6 months before bottling.

HERB LIQUEURS

Herbal liqueurs use alcohol or brandy as a base. There is no attempt to produce alcohol from the ingredients themselves by fermentation. The liqueurs may be left undistilled, in which case they remain more or less herb-flavored brandy, or they may be distilled to produce a "real" liqueur. This is, of course, the professional method of liqueur making, but it requires the use of a still or chemical retort, which is a little too elaborate and demanding for most people. However, I give an example of both types of liqueur making, the simple and the more complex, for those who are interested:

Simple Herb Liqueur

1 ounce fresh angelica stems or
   your favorite sweet herb (fennel,
   hyssop, rosemary, woodruff, balm,
   thyme, lemon verbena, marjoram,
   orange mint, lavender flowers)
1 pinch ground cloves and/or nutmeg
1 ounce bitter almonds
2 pints brandy (cooking brandy will do)

Chop the angelica or the other freshly gathered herb or herbs of your choice, and steep them in the brandy for 5 days with spices and the skinned and mashed bitter almonds. At the end of this time, strain the liquid through a fine mesh to remove all solid particles; a piece of muslin known as a Hippocrates sleeve in winemaking is usually recommended, but actually any thin untinted piece of muslin inside a funnel or strainer, or even a nylon stocking will do just as well. Before bottling, add about 2 cups liquid sugar (1 cup white sugar dissolved in 1 cup water), more or less according to how sweet you like your liqueurs.

Distilled Herb Liqueur

This is the recipe traditionally used for the composition of chartreuse liqueur. The bizarre ingredient measurements are the result of translation from the Continental European metric system. However, they are proportional and may be varied as required.

10½ ounces fresh hyssop leaves	⅔ ounce mace
10½ ounces fresh balm leaves	⅔ ounce saffron
5⅓ ounces fresh angelica leaves	5½ quarts potable wine alcohol
2⅙ ounces cinnamon	2⅝ cups white sugar

Steep all the ingredients except the sugar in the alcohol for 1 week, then distill. Sweeten the distillation with the sugar before bottling.

HERB CORDIALS

Cordials were simply beverages often but not invariably made with diluted wine or spirits, and flavored with herbs, spices, or syrups. By this definition today's vermouth cassis could be called a cordial. So could a vodka and tonic for that matter, or a cup of punch or Christmas wassail. The word itself means "comforting the heart," which could connote anything from a drink of welcome and cheer to a potion suitable for settling the digestion. In either instance, it is the alcohol involved which is the operative factor. In fact, by this definition most traditional herbal beverages of an alcoholic nature turn out to be cordials.

Another name for a cordial one often encounters in old herbals is hippocras. This derives from the thin muslin net, or Hippocrates sleeve, mentioned above, used to filter out the solid ingredients. "Philter" is another word used, but generally in a medicinal context.

Here is a selection of traditional cordials, alcoholic and nonalcoholic.

Absinthe Wine

A bitter and aromatic, not to say potent, wine, made from wormwood and herbs. This may be drunk mulled in winter.

2 teaspoons dried peppermint leaves	2 teaspoons dried wormwood
2 teaspoons dried thyme	2 teaspoons dried lavender
2 teaspoons dried hyssop	2 teaspoons dried marjoram
2 teaspoons dried sage	2 pints port wine

Steep the herbs in the wine for 1 week before filtering through muslin and bottling.

Angelica Wine

A sweet and delicious accompaniment to desserts:

> ¼ ounce fresh angelica leaves and stems, chopped
> 1 pinch ground nutmeg
> 1 quart white, red, or rosé wine
> 1 shot brandy
> White sugar

Steep the chopped angelica and the nutmeg in the wine for 2 days. Filter, and add the brandy and extra sugar to taste.

Balm Claret Cup

A refreshing drink for any hot day:

> 1 bottle light red wine
> 1 sprig fresh balm
> 3 or 4 fresh borage leaves
> 1 orange, sliced
> ½ cucumber, sliced thickly
> 1 ounce white sugar
> 1 shot brandy
> 2 cups soda water

Mix the ingredients together in an earthenware, ceramic, or glass jug (traditionally, with a silver spoon). Chill in the refrigerator for a couple of hours, and add 2 cups soda water and ice before serving.

Old-style Hippocras

This is a hippocras recipe attributed to the thirteenth-century Spanish alchemist and physician Arnald de Villeneuve, a pioneer, interestingly enough, in early research into the medicinal uses of what was then known as spirits of wine, but today as brandy!

> 3 ounces raisins
> 3 ounces ground nutmeg
> 3 ounces cloves
> 3 ounces cubebs (*Cubeba officinalis*)
> 3 liters (5¼ pints) red wine

Tie the raisins, nutmeg, cloves, and cubebs up in a cheesecloth bouquet and simply simmer it and the wine in an enamel pan until the wine has reduced to 2 liters (about 2½ pints). Add sugar to taste before serving in a punch bowl garnished with orange slices.

Alternatively, Arnald advises using:

> 3 ounces cinnamon
> 3 ounces ginger
> 3 ounces grains paradise
> 3 ounces cloves
> 1 pinch musk (use 1 drop
>   artificial essential oil here)

Again, simmer the wine down to ⅔ the original amount and add sugar to taste before serving.

New-style Hippocras

An ideal drink for the winter party:
Make a bouquet of:

> 4 teaspoons ground ginger
> 2 teaspoons ground nutmeg
> 2 tablespoons cinnamon
> 2 cloves
> Rinds of 2 oranges

Simmer the spices in 2 cups water mixed with 3 cups sugar for 10 minutes. Pour in 2 quarts red, white, or rosé wine, and heat until the surface turns creamy. Allow the spices to simmer for 20 minutes longer before removing them and serving in a punch bowl with a couple of sprigs of rosemary floating on top.

Hydromel

Another old-time herbal drink in the category of mead and hippocras is hydromel. As the name suggests, its primary constituents are water and honey.

1 ounce elder flowers	1 cup brandy
½ ounce orris root	3½ ounces honey
1 ounce crushed almonds	1 quart water

Steep the elder flowers, orris root (the dried root of the *Iris florentina*, obtainable from any herbal mail-order company), and almonds in the brandy for 3 days. Separately dissolve the honey in the warmed water, and add the brandy and herbs. Filter, cover, and leave in a warm place for 2 weeks. Filter once more before bottling.

Juniper Wine

This is a mysteriously piney-tasting cordial, with a hint of the *rezinas* of Greece and the fragrance of gin.

> 1 ounce juniper berries, crushed
> ½ teaspoon crushed coriander seeds
> 1 quart red or white wine
> 9 tablespoons white sugar
> 1 teaspoon vanilla extract

Steep the juniper berries and the coriander seeds in the cold wine for 24 hours. Add the sugar and the vanilla, stirring well until they are dissolved, and filter.

Mint Ale

A good drink for a hot day to match the Balm Claret Cup:

¼ cup spearmint leaves	1 tablespoon white sugar
¼ cup apple mint leaves	1 bottle ginger beer or ginger ale
2 cups boiling water	1 sprig of spearmint,
Juice of ½ lemon	orange mint or apple mint
Juice of ½ orange	

Infuse the spearmint and apple mint leaves for 15 minutes in the boiling water. Strain, and add the lemon and orange juice and the sugar. Mix well and chill in the refrigerator. Serve with the ginger beer or ale, ice, and the extra mint as garnish.

Sassafras Syrup

Simmer 3 ounces sassafras in 2 quarts distilled water for 15 minutes, strain, and add 1½ pints honey and 3½ pints molasses. Bring to a boil once more and stir in 1 tablespoon cream of tartar and allow to cool. Decant into sterilized bottles, cork tightly, and store for 24 hours in a cool place before using. Dilute with soda water and serve with ice cubes.

Woodruff Wine

The famous Maybowl recipe drunk on May 1 in Germany, the ancient pagan feast of Beltane, is an easy and delicious method of improving an indifferent white wine for any occasion:

> ½ ounce dried woodruff leaves
> 1 lemon, sliced
> 1 gallon white wine

Infuse the woodruff and the lemon in the wine for 4 to 6 hours (or longer if required). Filter and chill before serving.

Waldmeisterschnapps

Dried woodruff can also be steeped in brandy for a day or two to produce Waldmeisterschnapps, another old German favorite. A little sugar-cane syrup may also be added to sweeten it into a liqueur.

HERBAL TEAS

Finally, here is a selection of popular and time-honored herbal tisanes, or teas with which to finish off your meal. Herb teas are often advocated as good substitutes for coffee or for regular Indian or China tea. Not only do they promote the digestion, but while still acting in a mildly stimulating or calmative manner, they often lack the exaggerated amounts of theine or caffeine present in regular tea or coffee. They are therefore ideal for people who like to drink a hot beverage late at night but have trouble sleeping if they take tea or coffee.

Morning and Afternoon Teas

The following herbs are suitable for pleasant-tasting and stimulating morning and afternoon teas. They should be prepared as you would regular teas, adding sugar, honey, lemon, or milk to taste:

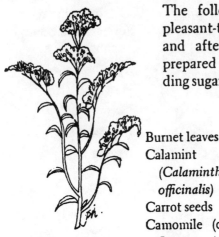

BLUE MOUNTAIN TEA,
or GOLDENROD
(*Solidago canadensis*)

Agrimony leaves
Anise seeds
Balm leaves
Basil leaves
Bay leaves
Bee-balm leaves (bergamot herb, oswego tea)
Betony (flavor with orange peel, lemon peel, or cloves)
Birch bark (*Betula lenta*)
Blackberry leaves (*Rubus fructicosus*)
Blackthorn berries (*Prunus spinosa*)
Buchu leaves (*Barosma crenata*)

Burnet leaves
Calamint leaves (*Calamintha officinalis*)
Carrot seeds
Camomile (common) flowers (*Anthemis nobilis*)
Chrysanthemum flowers
Costmary leaves (steep for 3 minutes)
Elecampane root (steep for 30 minutes)
Fenugreek seeds
Ginger root with cloves or nutmeg
Golden thyme
Guarana seeds (these contain about twice as much caffeine as coffee or tea)
Goldenrod herb (Blue Mountain tea)
Hawthorn leaves and berries
Juniper berries
Lavender flowers

Lemon grass and cloves
Lemon-scented thyme leaves
Licorice root
Marigold flowers
Mugwort leaves (steep for only 3 minutes)
Orange flowers
Orange bergamot or lemon mint leaves
Oregano leaves and tops
Peppermint leaves
Raspberry leaves
Red clover flowers
Rosemary leaves and tops
Rose hips
Sage leaves (good with mace, cinnamon, or melissa)
Savory leaves
Silver thyme
Spearmint leaves
Strawberry leaves
Sumac berries
Slippery-elm bark
Thyme leaves and tops
Violet flowers

Wintergreen leaves (*Gaultheria procumbens*)
Woodruff leaves
Yarrow flowers and tops

Yerba maté leaves (Paraguay tea or *Ilex paraguayensis;* drink with lemon and burned sugar)

Yerba santa leaves (*Eriodictyon glutinosum* and *E. californicum*)

Evening Teas

Fragrant tisanes to relax you and help you sleep can be composed out of the following herbs:

Catnip leaves
Camomile flowers (goes well with fennel seeds)
Elder flowers
Fennel seeds

Fraxinella leaves (*Dictamnus albus*)
German camomile (*Matricaria chamomilla*)
Hops flowers

Horehound leaves
Lime-tree flowers (linden)
Pennyroyal leaves
Primrose flowers
Verbena leaves

TRADITIONAL HERBAL TEA BLENDS

British Herb Tea

Dating from 1839, this herbal tisane was promoted as a substitute for Indian tea, being recommended to those anxious to avoid the stimulant action of theine, the active principle in the tea plant. The use of hawthorn leaves in tisanes is a very old European one, still popular among the Germans and French.

> 2 parts dried hawthorn leaves (*Crataegus oxyacantha*)
> 1 part dried sage leaves
> 1 part dried balm leaves

Mix well and prepare as you would regular tea, using 1 teaspoon for each cup.

Rose Tea

Another popular English tisane.

> 5 ounces dried red rosebuds,
>   or 5 ounces dried dog rose leaves
> 2 ounces dried balm
> 1 ounce dried rosemary

Prepare as above.

Meadowsweet Tea

For those who would prefer a more complex blend, here is an old rural tea redolent of summer fields:

1 ounce dried meadowsweet herb	1 ounce dried agrimony
1 ounce dried balm	¼ ounce dried rosebuds
1 ounce dried tormentil	¼ ounce dried primrose flowers
(Potentilla Tormentilla)	¼ ounce dried black currant leaves
1 ounce dried marjoram	(Ribes nigrum)

Prepare as above.

Wild Thyme Tea

A stimulant tea with a Mediterranean fragrance that calls for two types of thyme, the wild and the garden variety.

Take equal parts of:

Wild thyme	Sage	Hyssop
(Thymus serpyllum)	Rosemary	Peppermint
Garden thyme	Wormwood	Marjoram

Prepare as above.

Balm Tea

Another traditional and stimulant tea can be prepared with balm. Take and mix equal parts of:

Balm leaves
Rosemary
Lavender
Spearmint
Cloves

Sarsaparilla Tea

An early American favorite.
Mix:

1 part sassafras bark *(Sassafras officinalis)*
1 part licorice root *(Liquiritia officinalis)*
1 part sarsaparilla root *(Aralia nudicaulis)*
(optional)
½ part Virginian snakeroot *(Aristolochia Serpentaria,*
   the very same herb mentioned by Crateuas the Rhizotomist during the first century B.C.)

Allow 10 minutes for the tea to steep in a covered pot, 1
teaspoon herbs to each cup. If you like a bitter tonic edge to your
tea, add the Virginian snakeroot; otherwise omit. Sweeten with
honey, molasses, or sugar in any case. To experience what original
"root beer" once tasted like, substitute wintergreen leaves for the
snakeroot. It's delicious.

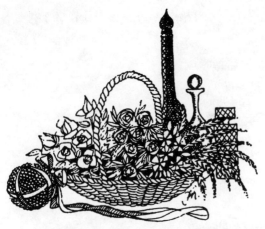

HERBAL PERFUMES AND INCENSES

HERBS AND SPICES WERE ONCE valued as highly for their perfume as for their curative properties. Indeed, the majority of perfume ingredients were once herbally derived. The importance of perfume is a fundamental one. Like a colorful precious stone or a fine piece of cloth, a perfume has obvious worth. If it looks or smells good, then it is good. Moreover, by adorning oneself with it, one can borrow its attractiveness and maybe even capture some of that "worth" for oneself. The biblical use of perfumed oils to anoint someone important as a token of esteem is a good example of this belief. A perfume worn by a person therefore has two primary functions: first, to please the wearer and make him or her feel good; and, second, to please other people and thereby render the wearer worthy, attractive, or desirable in their eyes.

Perfumes begin by simply smelling good. They become kingly or erotic only later by association. In today's culture, perfumes have become conventional stylized signals. If you wear perfume, you're out to turn someone on. If a woman wears musk or ambergris she generally means business. The same goes for the man who uses a cologne containing civet, patchouli, or vetivert, or so advertising campaigns would lead us to believe. We've come a long way from the simple, spicy aftershaves of the fifties, or the heliotrope perfume of the Victorians.

184

Today's perfumes may be broadly categorized under three headings. The "asexual" or "virginal" type of fragrance, nondescript, often used in household products, soaps, and bath salts, usually conveying the idea of cleanliness, purity, and so on. These are the light and airy perfumes, the citrons especially and the mints, lavender, raspberry, strawberry, and cinnamon. Then there are the "masculine" scents, sophisticated and aggressive, sometimes spicy, like clove, or woodsy like coumarin, pine, and civet, or bitter, like "Russian leather," bitter orange, and patchouli. The "feminine" fragrances are the sensual, and powerful, exotic essential oils derived from flowers such as rose and jasmine, and the old-time favorites of courtesans, such as musk, ambergris, and sandalwood.

These three perfume categories—"masculine," "feminine," and "neutral"—are really all that are left of a very ancient method of "type casting" dating from the early days of astrology in Babylon and ancient Egypt, but developed into a complicated science first by the Greeks and then by the Arabian occult philosophers, and finally by those of Renaissance Europe, like Marsilio Ficino and Tommaso Campanella. The theory goes something like this: Man's destiny, and indeed that of everything on earth, is controlled by the movements of the stars and planets. Ancient Egyptian and Babylonian priests worked out very precise charts of the motions of these heavenly bodies, and both they and the kings and pharaohs they ministered to lived their lives in strict accordance with what the stars foretold. If the pattern made by the stars one day was an unlucky one, then no great matters of state would be embarked upon that day. The most important astronomical bodies in the priests' calculations were the five planets that they knew—the five Wandering Lords, they called them—and the sun and moon. These seven movable celestial objects were known, and still are, as the seven "planets" of astrology: Saturn, Jupiter, Mars, the sun, Venus, Mercury, and the moon. Now each of these planets was thought to exert a particular type of influence upon daily life when it was overhead in the sky; it had a peculiar character of its own, in fact. Saturn, the old Greco-Roman god of time, was a stern judge, and brought a grim, "Saturnine," and oppressive influence to bear on matters. Jupiter, on the other hand, the old ruler of Olympus, brought feasting and jollity, a "Jovial" influence. Mars the soldier brought strife or courage in his wake, depending on his aspect. The sun was resplendent and regal, and gave help in arts, sciences, and medicine, for his character was that of Apollo, the sun god, whose special province these matters were. Venus was the goddess of love and beauty, and Mercury the god of messengers and merchants. The lady moon Diana had three sides to her character: she was a virgin huntress, a fertile Mother Goddess, and the queen of the dead, depending on which quarter she appeared in, new moon, full moon, or dark of the moon.

These "planets," therefore, all became convenient pigeonholes in which to categorize things. Graveyards and prisons corresponded to Saturn. Jupiter ruled feasting and hunting, Venus cosmetics, and so on. Colors were likewise attributed to them. Saturn governed black, Jupiter blue, Mars red, the sun golden-yellow, Venus green, Mercury brown or a mixture of colors, the moon silver or white. Perfumes were also pigeonholed: Saturn ruled all bitter and mournful perfumes, like myrrh and cypress—cypress trees grow in cemeteries and myrrh was once used to embalm the dead, both of which associations strengthen the link to Saturn. In fact, psychological association is the key to this whole process.

Jupiter ruled cloves, nutmeg, and saffron, spices used extensively in cooking and therefore associated with feasting. Mars governed aggressive and suggestively warlike smells like gunpowder and hot iron. Very few of his odors are suitable for perfume, except pine and fir oils. The sun ruled frankincense, the deity offering of pagan and Christian faiths alike, and bay, the favorite tree of Apollo; Venus the rose, the myrtle, and the violet, age-old feminine perfumes; Mercury lavender and marjoram, intellectual and asexual fragrances, cinnamon and citrus fruits, all used extensively around the house and in commerce; the chaste moon governed night-blooming flowers, virginal lilies and camphor gum, a substance that produces a feeling of numbing cold when applied locally to the skin, and has a calming and soothing effect when used internally, although paradoxically it is used to stimulate the heart in cases of heart failure.

Marsilio Ficino was a fifteenth-century physician who took over this old astrological lore from the Arabians and brought it up to date. He maintained in his widely read book on astrological medicine, *De Vita coelitus comparanda*, that since we were so heavily influenced by the planets, we should be well advised to surround ourselves with beneficial astrological colors and substances, which included perfumes ruled by the "cheerful" and "lucky" planets, Jupiter, Venus, Mercury, and, above all, the sun. All herbs in ancient times had been thought to be ruled by the stars, but here was a practical and updated version of the theory: astrological perfumes! In the seventeenth century, herbalists like William Coles poured scorn upon the practice of blending astrology with herbalism. However, they still clung to the notion that the aroma of herbs could be in some way beneficial to people. John Gerard said, "The savor or smell of the water-mint rejoyceth the heart of man." Of the meadowsweet he said, "The smell thereof makes the heart merrie and joyful and delighteth the senses," and of rosemary, "It comforteth the brain, the memorie, the inward senses and comforteth the heart and maketh it merry." Ficino and Culpeper, and for that matter any astrologer-herbalist, would claim that the mints were ruled by Venus, meadowsweet by Jupiter, and rosemary by the sun, and this is the reason for their being so beneficial. Gerard does not say as much, and Coles and his more rationalist colleagues would vigorously deny it. They had thrown out the theory but paradoxically retained the practice. The practice was, after all, what counted. Fine aromas do indeed make you feel good. It is an undeniable psychological fact, however you wish to explain it. Astrology in this its most rudimentary aspect was, after all, simply a poetic scale that enabled one to classify and identify broad areas of human experience.

As you can see, today's perfume categories have shrunk from seven quite specifically defined ones to three rather general ones. The "masculine" planets, Saturn, Jupiter, Mars, and the sun, have donated their odors to men's colognes, aftershaves, and deodorants, and the "feminine" plants, Venus and the moon, to women's perfumes. Mercury, considered an androgynous entity by the ancient astrologers, has filled in any gaps left by the others, providing "cover" scents rather than perfumes which stand on their own.

Most present-day herbalists do not subscribe to the old astrological theories, even when it is only a matter of perfume blending. Many seem anxious not to become involved in what they regard as the crank occult fringe, possibly being only too aware that a considerable portion of the population would have up until quite recently regarded any herbalist as a crank or faddist. Respectability,

188 / MASTERING HERBALISM

especially with the Food and Drug Administration and the American Medical Association breathing down your neck, is a much sought-after thing, apparently. I am not advocating a return to Culpeper's astrological medicine, but I do feel there was more than an element of truth in the old astrological notions regarding the psychological categorizing of herbal fragrances. Today sachets and potpourris are for the most part made for purely practical purposes as deodorants and moth repellents, which I think is a great shame. There is much more to our sense of smell than this rather limited approach.

For those who do wish to consider their herbs astrologically, however, I give a planetary catalog of herbs and spices in Chapter 6.

Sachets and Potpourris

The easiest way to employ herbal fragrance is in a sachet or potpourri. Sachets are little bags of highly scented aromatic herbs and spices. Once people carried them about on their persons, although today cologne has replaced them in this area. They are, however, still used to perfume linen closets and keep the moths out, and they make delightful gifts at Yule. A jar of fragrant herbs and spices kept about the house for its perfume's sake alone is known as a potpourri. Sachets and potpourris in fact are practically interchangeable terms.

Today most commercially available sachets and potpourris are heavily perfumed with artificial floral essences. Any homemade sachet of your own will usually be far superior in quality. For one thing, you can choose your own ingredients, and, for another, you can make quite sure allergenic chemicals are not incorporated. Needless to say, you also get the chance to be truly creative rather than to buy your pleasure ready-made. A sachet or potpourri can be anything from a simple collection of dried fragrant leaves and petals from your garden to an involved mixture of herbs, spices, and oils, carefully balanced and blended according to your own or a traditional formula over a long period of time. You may find that when you start formulating sachet mixes of your own you will have an overwhelming desire to innovate and explore new combinations. Go right ahead. The secret of perfume-making—and this applies to sachets too—is to find fragrances that "click" together, that is, "interlock" to form a third, totally new scent. If they do not click, you will still have two separate and quite distinguishable perfumes. "That smells like peppermint and roses," will be an outsider's comment here rather than, "That's fantastic! How did you make it?"

A sachet or a potpourri contains three basic types of ingredients:

1. An agent, or primary scent, often in liquid form;

2. A base, or secondary scent, sometimes called a blender, usually an herb;

3. A fixative, generally a resin, wood, or root.

The agent and the base are the two scents mentioned earlier which have to click together. The fixative, often a comparatively neutral-smelling resin, is added to cement the union. Floral essential oils are often used as agents and, though powerful, they are volatile and evaporate quickly, leaving you with your secondary ingredient. However, if a harmonious fixative is added, it will absorb the agent and incorporate its perfume in its own, thus extending its short life considerably. A well-made sachet or potpourri can in fact retain its potency for up to thirty or forty years.

There are literally innumerable sachet and potpourri recipes in existence. Every handwritten "still-room book," descendant of the old herbal, halfway between a family cookbook and a home doctor, usually contains dozens of personal favorites of the master or lady of the household. Many of them require ingredients now difficult or impossible to obtain, like real musk and ambergris, or else in such vast quantities as could be expected only from the owners of palatial country estates. However, this need not trouble you. Once you understand the principle behind sachet making, you can go ahead and invent your own. There are of course many tried and true combinations of herbs and spices, such as roses and sandalwood, or orris root and anise seed, and so on, some of which I shall list later.

Before going any further, here is a fairly complete list of most if not all of the sachet and potpourri ingredients you can buy today. Many of them you can grow or collect yourself. Several of them you may have already on your kitchen shelf. Before you start buying essential oils, try a few drops of your favorite cologne as a starter. Some herb companies and pharmacies market their own special brands of essential oil, or even blends which they sell under a simple flower name, like Heliotrope Oil. However, when I list an oil, I refer only to the plain herbal or floral essence. Many of the fragrances are available in both herb or essential oil form. The latter is the most powerful, and is best used as an agent. Use the herb as a base.

SPICY SCENTS

Allspice berries (also known as pimiento or Jamaica pepper; smells like a mixture of cloves, nutmeg, and cinnamon)
Canella wood (smells like cinnamon)
Cassia wood, buds or oil (smells like cinnamon)
Cinnamon bark or oil
Cloves, whole, ground, or oil
Cubebs (smell a little like mace)
Galangal oil (sweet, spicy fragrance; the root itself doesn't have much scent)
Ginger root or oil
Mace blades
Nigella seeds (warm, spicy smell)
Nutmeg, ground, or oil
Nutmeg geranium leaves

SWEET AND FLORAL SCENTS

Acacia flowers
Ambergris oil or tincture (very sweet and rarely used alone; use the artificial variety, as the real is prohibitively expensive)
Apple blossoms or oil
Apple mint leaves
Bois de rose oil
Cactus flowers or oil
Calamus root or oil (also known as sweet flag, this has a pleasant fruity fragrance)
Campernella oil (smells like jonquil)
Cardamom pods or oil (very aromatic when crushed)
Carnation flowers or oil
Champac oil (a variety of magnolia)
Cherry blossoms or oil
Clove pink flowers or oil
Clover flowers or oil
Coriander seeds (pungently sweet when crushed)
Frangipani flowers or oil
Gardenia flowers or oil
Geranium leaves or oil
Guaiac wood oil (roselike fragrance)
Heliotrope flowers or oil (like a mixture of anise, almond, and vanilla)
Honeysuckle flowers or oil
Hyacinth flowers or oil
Jasmine flowers or oil
Lavender flowers or oil
Lilac flowers or oil
Lily flowers or oil
Lily of the valley flowers or oil

Linden flowers (*Tilia europaea*, also known as lime flowers)

Lotus flowers or oil

Magnolia flowers or oil

Mignonette flowers (*Reseda odorata*)

Mimosa flowers or oil

Narcissus flowers or oil (also known as jonquil)

Neroli oil (also known as bitter orange flower oil; generally this is extremely expensive, but there are many good blends and synthetics on the market)

Neroli petalae oil (sweet orange flower oil; about half the price of true neroli)

Nicotiana flowers or oil

Night-scented stock flowers or oil

Orange mint leaves

Orris root or oil (the root of the iris; it has a strong violet fragrance)

Palmarosa oil (geraniumlike fragrance)

Peach blossom flowers or oil

Pineapple mint leaves (very good in sachets)

Raspberry leaves or oil (mildly fragrant leaves)

Rosebuds, petals, or oil (rose attar is one of the most expensive essential oils on the market, costing retail upward of $1000 per pound! Use one of the substitute oils or blends.)

Rose geranium leaves (an excellent substitute for rosebuds, in some cases even more fragrant)

Rosemary leaves or oil

Spike lavender flowers or oil (smell like an herby blend of camphor and lavender)

Strawberry leaves or oil

Stephanotis flowers or oil

Sweetbriar leaves

Sweet pea flowers or oil

Syringa blossoms or oil

Tuberose oil

Tulip flowers or oil

Violet leaves or oil (ionone is the inexpensive artificial violet oil used in most violet-scented perfumes)

Wallflower flowers or oil

Wisteria flowers or oil

Yarrow flowers

Ylang-ylang flowers or oil (very powerful and exotic)

Yucca flowers

CITRUS SCENTS

Balm leaves

Bergamot leaves or oil (a variety of orange)

Bigarade, oil of (bitter or Seville orange peel oil)

Citronella oil

Gas plant leaves (fraxinella)

Grapefruit leaves, peel, or flowers

Lemongrass

Lemon leaves, peel, or flowers

Lemon oil (extracted from the peel)

Lemon-scented geranium leaves

Lemon verbena leaves

Lime leaves, peel, and flowers (*Citrus acida*)

Lime oil (extracted from the peel)

Orange leaves, peel, and flowers

Orange oil (extracted from the peel)

Pettigrain, oil of (orange leaf oil)

Portugal, oil of (sweet orange peel oil)

Tangerine leaves, peel, and flowers

Perilla leaves (aniselike fragrance)

Saffron filaments or oil

Sage leaves or oil

Spearmint leaves or oil

Sweet cicely leaves, seeds, or oil (a myrrhlike fragrance)

Tansy leaves

Thyme leaves or oil

Wintergreen leaves or oil

Woodruff leaves (smell like new-mown hay)

HERBY SCENTS

Angelica root or oil

Anise leaves, seeds, or oil

Basil leaves or oil (clovelike fragrance)

Calamint leaves

Costmary leaves (a mixture of mint and chrysanthemum fragrance)

Dill seed or oil

Dittany of Crete leaves (a little like the smell of dried, as opposed to fresh, marjoram)

Fennel seeds or oil

Marjoram leaves or oil (the oil is much more fragrant than the dried leaves)

Oregano leaves or oil (wild marjoram)

Pennyroyal leaves or oil (somewhere in between peppermint and vanilla)

Peppermint-scented geranium leaves

Peppermint leaves or oil

WOODSY SCENTS

Acacia wood and oil (needs reinforcing by other fragrances)

Almond oil, sweet

Ambretta seeds (also known as amber and musk seed)

Ambrosia (also known as chenopodium or wormseed; smells a little like eucalyptus)

Balm of Gilead (poplar buds; very sweet, mellow scent)

Bayberry bark or oil

Bay leaves or oil

Birch bark or oil

Brazilwood (shows up in some old recipes; nothing really exciting)

Cajeput oil (smells like a delicious combination of rosemary, camphor, and cardamom)

Camphor, gum

Cascarilla bark (used a lot in incense recipes, too)

Cedarwood chips, raspings, leaves, or oil

Chenopodium (see ambrosia)

Civet oil or tincture (like rose attar and ambergris, civet is extremely expensive; use a synthetic or blend)

Clary sage leaves and oil (smells like balsam of tolu)

Deer's tongue leaves (strong, vanillalike fragrance)

Eucalyptus leaves or oil

Frankincense, gum or oil (also known as olibanum)

Juniper oil

Labdanum leaves

Lignum aloes (*Aquilaria agallocha* only; do not buy bitter aloes or aloes socrotine by mistake)

Mastic, gum (must be combined with an oil)

Melilot flowers (smells like tonka or woodruff, being rich in coumarin)

Musk oil or tincture (useful in practically any perfume; use artificial or blended variety)

Musk-scented geranium leaves

Myrtle leaves (faint eucalyptus fragrance)

Oak moss (very woodsy)

Pine needles or oil

Rhodium oil (wood of Rhodes oil)

Sandalwood raspings or oil (white or yellow; the red is a different wood altogether and is used only in dyeing)

Sandarac, gum (cedarwood gum; must be combined with an oil)

Sassafras wood or oil (spicy and woodsy)

Spruce oil

Sumbul root (also known as musk root; delightful musky scent)

Sweet fern (woodsy)

Sweet gale leaves (*Myrica gale*)

Thus, gum (spruce or pine resin; must be combined with an oil)

Tonka beans (vanillalike aroma)

Vanilla pods or essence

Vetivert (also known as khus-khus; fabulous fragrance like myrrh and sandalwood)

Walnut leaves (no real fragrance to speak of, but they sometimes turn up in old recipes)

Wormseed (see ambrosia)

BITTER OR PUNGENT SCENTS

Almond oil, bitter

Caraway seeds or oil (often used in old sachet recipes)

Catnip leaves or oil

Cotton lavender leaves

Cypress leaves, roots, or oil

Galbanum, gum (must be combined with an oil)

Hyssop leaves or oil (the oil is more fragrant than the dried leaf)

Life everlasting leaves

Myrrh, gum (must be combined with an oil)

Opopanax, gum (must be combined with an oil)

Patchouli leaves or oil (a gorgeous "earthy" fragrance)

Rue leaves or oil (use these carefully; see Rue entry in Chapter 1)

Santolina leaves (another variety of lavender cotton)

Southernwood leaves (bitter, lemony smell)

Wormwood leaves or oil (bitter)

FIXATIVES

(General formula for sachets and potpourris: 1 ounce fixative to every 2 quarts herbs.)

Ambergris oil or tincture

Asafoetida, gum (this should be used only in a highly purified form in "Oriental" perfumes; the regular resin has a pungently offensive odor)

Balsam of Peru (extremely useful; can be used as a fixative for practically all sachets; particularly good for heliotrope, linden, and lotus)

Balsam of tolu (again, extremely useful, especially so for ambretta, acacia, champac, honeysuckle, magnolia, wallflower, and any dry potpourris)

Benzoin, gum (another handy favorite, also known in old herbals as gum Benjamin)

Calamus root or oil

Castoreum

Cedarwood chips or oil (use sparingly, as it is very powerful)

Chenopodium

Civet oil or tincture

Clary sage

Lemon peel

Mastic, gum

Musk oil or tincture

Opopanax, gum

Orange peel

Orris root

Patchouli leaves

Sandalwood (useful for any rose mixture)

Sandarac, gum

Storax, gum (also known as stacte in old recipes)

Sumbul root

Tangerine peel

Thus, gum (both pine and spruce resin go by this name now; it used to be another name for frankincense)

Vetivert

SACHET AND POTPOURRI HERBS USED FOR THEIR SHAPE OR COLOR

Alkanet flowers (blue)
Bachelor's buttons (yellow)
Bee balm flowers (red)
Borage flowers (blue)
Broom flowers (yellow)
Camomile flowers (yellow)
Cardinal flowers (red)
Cornflower heads or petals (blue)
Daisies (white, pink, blue)
Delphinium flowers (blue)
Elecampane flowers (yellow)
Hibiscus flowers (red or pink)
Hollyhock flowers (pink, red, white, or purple)
Jasmine flowers (white)
Larkspur flowers (pink, purple, or blue)
Lavender flowers (blue)
Mallow flowers (pink, purple, or white)

Marigold flowers or petals (*Calendula*; yellow or orange)
Melilot flowers (yellow or white)
Mullein flowers (white or yellow)
Nasturtium flowers (red, orange, or yellow)
Pansy flowers (variegated blue, purple, yellow, and white)
Primrose flowers (white, yellow, red or purple)
Purple basil leaves (purple)
Rosebuds (generally pink)
Rosemary flowers (blue)
Rose petals (dark red, pink, and occasionally white are commercially available in dried form; of course, if you grow your own . . .)
Safflower flowers (red)
Tansy flowers (yellow)
Violet flowers (purple)

If you wish to dry your own garden flowers, retaining their shape and as much of their color as possible, fill a small cake tin a quarter full of salt or fine washed and dried sand and place the flower or flowers upon it. Now gently sprinkle the flowers with more salt or sand, taking care not to crush the petals, until the flowers are completely submerged. Leave the cake tin in the sun for several days, or for a short time in an oven at low heat. Remove the flowers gently and dust off the sand or salt before storing them in plastic bags or airtight boxes.

MAKING A SACHET

Gather together your ingredients: the dried herb and spice base, the essential oil agent, and the fixative. Grind the herbs, spices, and fixative to a coarse powder in a mill or a pestle and mortar. This process was known to old-time herbalists as trituration. Add 1 drop of your essential oil now to half the powder, and mix it in thoroughly. Now take a good sniff and see if you like it. If you feel the agent is not strong enough, add another drop or two. Repeat the procedure for the remaining half of the powder before combining them. If, on the other hand, you find that 1 drop is too much, add the remainder of the base without any more agent. If it is *still* too powerful, mix up another batch of fixative and base and add it in. Be sure to keep track of your actions in note form, however, especially the proportions you use. When you come up with an exquisite fragrance after possibly considerable experimenting, you will feel justifiably irritated if you cannot repeat it again. When you have completed your sachet mix to your satisfaction, let it sit for a few days and mellow. Sometimes the fragrance takes time to blend. Then sew it up in a little cushion of thin muslin. For those without patience or aptitude with needle and thread, the smaller sizes of so-called small parts bags, obtainable from most companies specializing in mailing and wrapping materials, will do the job effectively. Failing that, a piece of cheesecloth tied up with ribbon will also work.

SOME TYPICAL SACHET RECIPES, ANCIENT AND MODERN

An Excellent Damask Powder [1]

"You may take of Rose leaves four ounces, cloves one ounce, lignum Rhodium [Rhodes wood] two ounces, Storax one ounce

[1] From *Ram's Little Dodoen* (1606).

and a halfe. Muske and Civet of each ten grains [about 1/6 tea-spoon]; beat and incorporate them well together."

Clove Pink Sachet

To compose a delicious carnation-smelling sachet, take:

1 ounce lavender flowers	1 teaspoon allspice
2 ounces powdered orris root	10 drops rose oil
½ ounce deer's tongue	10 drops lavender oil
½ ounce patchouli	10 drops neroli oil
2 teaspoons ground cloves	15 drops sandalwood oil

Triturate well.

"A perfume for a Sweet bagg" [2]

"Take half a pound of Cypress Roots, a pound of Orris, 3 quarters of a pound of Rhodium, a pound of Coriander Seed, 3 quarters of a pound of Calamus, 3 oranges stuck with cloves, 2 ounces of Benjamin [Benzoin], and an ounce of Storax and 4 pecks of Damask Rose leaves, a peck of dryed sweet Marjeram [Marjoram], a pretty stick of Juniper shaved very thin, some lemon pele dryed and a stick of Basil [Brazilwood]: let all these be powdered very grosely for ye first year and immediately put into your baggs; the next year pound and work it and it will be very good again."

A Heliotrope Sachet

Heliotrope was a favorite scent of the Victorians smelling like—well, try it and see . . .

20 parts powdered orris root	2½ parts cut vanilla bean
10 parts rosa centifolia buds or petals	⅟₁₀ part powdered musk
5 parts ground tonka bean	1 drop bitter almond oil

Pound musk and vanilla and add the other ingredients. Pass through a large sieve.

[2] From *Mary Doggett: Her Book of Receipts* (1682).

A Simple Heliotrope Sachet

Whereas the previous recipe approximated the fragrance of heliotrope by blending other essences, this one requires the real McCoy essential oil.

8 ounces powdered orris root
4 ounces damask rose petals
2 ounces ground tonka beans
½ ounce ground vanilla pods
⅛ ounce heliotrope oil

Note: Geranium leaves are sometimes substituted for the rose petals in some recipes.

"A Sweet Bag for Linen" [3]

"Take of Orris roots, sweet Calamus, cypress-roots, of dried Lemon-peel, and dried Orange-peel; of each a pound; a peck of dried roses; make all these into a gross powder; coriander-seed four ounces, nutmegs an ounce and a half, an ounce of cloves; make all these into fine powder and mix with the other; add musk and ambergris; then take four large handfuls of lavender flowers dried and rubbed; of sweet-marjoram, orange-leaves, and young walnut-leaves, of each a handful, all dried and rubbed; mix all together, with some bits of cotton perfumed with essences, and put it up into silk bags to lay with your linen."

A Verbena Sachet

Verbena was the favorite scent of Sarah Bernhardt. This is a particularly refreshing sachet.

4 ounces lemon verbena leaves   ¼ ounce bergamot oil
1 ounce caraway seed   ¼ ounce lemon oil
2 ounces orange peel   1 drop verbena oil
2 ounces lemon peel

Mix well together.

[3] From The Compleat Housewife (1736).

A Simple Lavender Sachet

Lavender flowers keep their perfume far longer if they are blended with a fixative as follows:

> 8 ounces lavender flowers
> 1½ ounces powdered benzoin gum
> A few drops lavender oil

Three Basic Rose Sachets

Rose is a very extensively used fragrance in sachet making.
1. Mix together

> 4 ounces sandalwood raspings,
> 8 ounces rose petals or buds, and
> 1 teaspoon rose oil.

2. Mix together

> 8 ounces rose petals or buds,
> 1 ounce rose geranium leaves,
> 4 ounces sandalwood raspings, and
> ⅛ ounce rose oil.

3. "A Bag to Smell unto for Melancholy, or to cause one to sleep:—Take drie Rose leaves [petals], keep them close in a glasse which will keep them sweet, then take powder of Mints, powder of Cloves in a grosse powder, and put the same to the Rose leaves, then put all these together in a bag, and take that to bed with you, and it will cause you to sleep, and it is good to smell unto at other times."

Frangipani Sachet I

Again an approximation this time of the scent of the frangipani blossom:

> 8 ounces powdered orris root
> ½ ounce vetivert
> ½ ounce sandalwood raspings
> ¼ teaspoon sandalwood oil
> ¼ teaspoon rose oil

Frangipani Sachet II

1 ounce vetivert
1 ounce sage leaves
1 ounce sandalwood raspings
12 ounces powdered orris root

⅛ teaspoon neroli oil
⅛ teaspoon rhodium oil
⅛ teaspoon sandalwood oil

An "Oriental" Sachet

2 ounces vetivert
2 ounces rosebuds
1 ounce patchouli leaves
1 ounce ground mace
A few drops rose oil

A Spice Sachet

You probably have most of the ingredients of this sachet already.

8 ounces powdered orris root
6 ounces sandalwood raspings
4 ounces lavender flowers
2 ounces patchouli leaves

1 ounce powdered cloves
½ ounce powdered allspice
¼ ounce powdered cinnamon
A few drops musk oil

Wildflower Sachet

This is a light, attractive fragrance. Its name is fully justified.

2 ounces lavender flowers
1 ounce marjoram
1 ounce caraway seed
2 ounces calamus root
¼ ounce ground cloves

1 ounce orange mint
2 ounces rosebuds or petals
½ ounce rosemary
1 ounce thyme
No essential oil needed here

A Traditional Moth-repellent Sachet

Sachets are of course, a time-honored method of discouraging moths. Not only do they make the clothes smell fragrant, but they are free from all toxic chemicals.

Mix equal portions of the following:

Dried lemon peel
Tansy
Rosemary
Lavender
Pennyroyal

Other traditional moth-repellent aromatics that may be made up into linen sachets are: camphor bark or gum, cassia bark, cedar-wood raspings or chips, camomile flowers, lavender cotton leaves, pyrethrum leaves, rue leaves, santolina leaves, sassafras chips, spearmint leaves, thyme, winter savory, and woodruff leaves. Winter savory and pennyroyal are both flea-banes too. Try putting a sachet of these herbs in your dog's bed. They certainly smell better than flea collars.

POMANDERS

The word "pomander" is really a corruption of two French words: *Pomme*, meaning apple, and *ambre*, meaning ambergris, a fatty substance obtained from the cachalot whale, which exudes a powerful fragrance similar to musk. It is used extensively in perfumery. Most pomanders, however, are made of citrus fruits rather than apples, oranges being the favorite. Nowadays they fulfill the same functions as linen sachets, but they also have a certain decorative medieval charm about them that's hard to resist and makes them handsome and traditional midwinter gifts for your friends.

Simply take an orange and stick it with as many cloves (sharp ends inward) as will fit, covering every inch of the surface so it resembles a little knobbly nut. Now roll the studded orange in a mixture of gum benzoin and orris root pounded fine with a little essential oil or perfume tincture of your choice added. (Musk, civet, and ambergris work superbly here, either singly or in combination.) Finally wrap your pomander in a sheet of tissue paper and store it for a month or two in a cool, dry place. When you wish to use it, dust it off, tie a brightly colored silk ribbon or yarn about it, and hang it in your clothes closet or wrap it as a gift.

Potpourris

There are two kinds of potpourri: the "dry" sort and the "wet" sort. The dry is the easier to make, but the wet is the most enduring.

DRY POTPOURRI

Simply gather your selected well-dried herbs, barks, and leaves together and mix them with the oils and spices in a large nonporous glass or ceramic bowl, keeping careful track of your measurements as you did in the sachet mix. When you achieve your desired perfume, add the fixative and various dried flowers of your choice for color. Mix well again, and pack the potpourri into your selected container or containers. Patterned china "rose jars" or "sweet jars" were used in the old days. However, the attractive transparent Italian glass jars available at most import stores make fine containers, for they allow you to see the potpourri through the glass. Cover tightly before storing.

Cypress-rose Mixture

2 ounces cypress root or leaves
2 ounces orris root
2 ounces calamus root
2 ounces dried orange peel
2 ounces dried lemon peel
1 ounce bruised coriander seeds
   (use a pestle and mortar for this)
1 quart rosebuds
2 ounces lavender flowers
½ ounce marjoram leaves

½ ounce walnut leaves
½ ounce lemon verbena leaves
½ ounce woodruff, melilot, or
   deer's tongue leaves
½ ounce ground cloves
½ ounce ground nutmeg
A few drops musk,
   civet, or patchouli
A few drops ambergris

Mix well and store in a closely covered jar for a week or two, stirring occasionally, before transferring to your potpourri jar.

A Spice Potpourri

4 ounces uniodized salt	¼ ounce powdered borax
4 ounces coarse salt	¼ ounce orris root (powdered)
¼ ounce cinnamon	¼ ounce chopped and dried orange peel
¼ ounce cloves	¼ ounce chopped and dried lemon peel
¼ ounce nutmeg	¼ teaspoon musk
¼ ounce allspice	or any other essential oil
¼ ounce gum benzoin	

Mix well and store in a tightly lidded jar for a week or two, stirring occasionally before transferring to your potpourri jar.

A Spice Base for Any Dry Potpourri

This handy formula can be incorporated with any of your homegrown herbs and flowers you wish to make into a dry potpourri.

To every 2 quarts of dried herbs, add:

1 teaspoon ground cloves	¼ teaspoon ground allspice
1 teaspoon ground mace	¼ teaspoon gum storax
1 teaspoon ground cinnamon	¼ teaspoon gum benzoin
¼ teaspoon bruised coriander seed	2 teaspoons powdered orris root

Simple Potpourri

2 ounces lavender flowers
2 ounces orris root
1 ounce ground rosemary
5 drops rose or any other essential oil

Mix well and store in a closely lidded jar for a week or two before transferring to the potpourri jar.

An English Rose Potpourri

4 cups dried rosebuds
¼ teaspoon dried
   rose geranium leaves
¼ teaspoon powdered orris root

¼ teaspoon ground cinnamon
¼ teaspoon ground allspice
¼ teaspoon dried orange mint

Mix well and store in a tightly lidded jar for a week or two before transferring to the potpourri jar.

Three Dry Potpourris

1. For a blend with a dark, old fragrance, mix:

Sandalwood
Patchouli
Deer's tongue
Rosebuds

Rose geranium
Lavender
Nutmeg
Cypress

2. For a sweeter, mellower mixture, use:

Calamus
Rose geranium
Lavender

Pine needles
Nutmeg
Lemon verbena

3. Finally, for a really fabulous perfume, mix:

Sandalwood
Rose geranium
Lavender
Sage

A Scottish Potpourri

Take all or any of these ingredients:

Dried rosebuds
Dried clove carnations
Dried lavender flowers
Dried woodruff flowers
Dried rosemary flowers
Dried violet flowers

Dried lemon verbena
(flowers
Dried bay leaves
Dried sweetbriar leaves
Dried balm leaves
Dried lemon leaves

Dried thyme
A little spearmint
Dried lemon peel
Dried orange peel
Dried tangerine peel

Mix the leaves and peel with:

½ pound kitchen salt	1 nutmeg, grated (about 1 teaspoon)
½ pound bay (coarse) salt	½ teaspoon ground cloves
½ ounce storax gum	½ teaspoon ground allspice
2 tablespoons ground orris root	1 ounce bergamot oil

Fill a tall jar with layers of the mixture interspersed with layers of the herbs and flowers. Close the jar tightly for a week or two, and mix from time to time. Then transfer to your decorative potpourri jar or jars.

WET POTPOURRIS

In wet potpourris the petals, flowers, and herbs should only be allowed to become wilted rather than completely dry. Consequently you will need to grow your own rather than order from a mail-order company. Whereas you can use jars or pots of any size or shape to prepare dry potpourris, the wet variety demands a rather straight jar with a tightly fitting or screw lid. A large mayonnaise or pickle jar will do fine.

Pick over your flower heads and petals first, removing as much of the stalks and green parts as you can. Don't worry about each flower's being a splendid specimen. They are going to be squashed into a shapeless mass anyway. Use any perfumed flower you have in your garden or yard—lavender, gardenia, carnation, whatever—and any aromatic herb or leaf you care to. Citrus peel, bay leaves, and any sweet-smelling herb in your cupboard can also be added. Be inventive. Don't use any spices, though; they come later. Now sprinkle the bottom of the jar with *coarse* kitchen salt (known as bay salt in old recipes). Kosher salt is fine for this. Add the partially dried leaves and flowers—they should have a flabby, leathery consistency—in a layer ½ inch deep. Then add more salt, then another layer of herbs and flowers, and so on. When you have exhausted your supply of ingredients, take a tumbler that will fit through the neck of the pickle jar, and ram all the herbs and flowers down mercilessly with the bottom of it. Don't use a metal can for this purpose, as metal reacts chemically with herbal essences and often spoils them. Add more wilted herbs and flower petals as you harvest them throughout the summer and keep interspersing them with salt layers and ramming them down firmly. At the end of 2 or 3 months you will have a moist, fragrant "pickle" in your jar. You are now ready for the final stage. Loosen the contents of the jar with the handle of a wooden spoon, and tip it out on a sheet of waxed paper. You will see that the petals and leaves have been squashed into a thick flaking cake. Break this up and mix it all well together. Now, to every 2 quarts of this mixture, add the following preparation:

1 tablespoon crushed cardamom
    seed
½ chopped dried orange rind
1 teaspoon ground allspice
1 teaspoon cinnamon
1 teaspoon ground cloves
1 teaspoon ground nutmeg

½ vanilla pod, crushed, or
    1 tablespoon dried deer's
    tongue leaves
1 ounce dry fixative
    (orris root or benzoin or
    a mixture of both)

Mix everything well together now, and toss in a few drops of essential oil of your choice if you wish to add extra zing. Musk, civet, and ambergris are good ones to try. Don't overdo them, though. Not more than 4 drops in all are needed. Finally, add some dried flowers for color, and pack your completed potpourri in decorative jars for placing about the house or giving away as gifts. When you wish to fill a room with its fragrance, simply lift the lid for a short period.

Devonshire Potpourri

Gather the following flowers in the morning when they are dry, and lay them in the sun until evening:

Roses
Orange flowers
Jasmine
Lavender

Do the same with smaller quantities of:

Thyme leaves
Bay leaves
Sage leaves
Marjoram leaves

Make a mixture of the following:

6 pounds bay (coarse) salt	2 ounces cinnamon	1 ounce rose otto (use rose oil)
4 ounces sandalwood	2 ounces cloves	1 teaspoon musk oil
4 ounces calamus root	4 ounces benzoin gum	½ ounce ground cardamom
4 ounces cassia buds	1 ounce storax gum	

Make alternate layers of the flowers and herbs with the salt and spice mixture in a tall jar, pressing them down firmly as you do. Keep for 3 months before using.

Rose Potpourri

Take fresh rose petals and pack them in a glass jar between layers of coarse salt. Continue to do this until the jar is filled, pressing down the petals each time you add more. When the jar is filled, leave it for 1 last week in a dry, cool place. Then spread the petals out on waxed paper and add the following spice mixture:

2 ounces powdered orris root	4 drops rose geranium oil
½ teaspoon ground mace	20 drops eucalyptus oil
½ teaspoon ground cloves	10 drops bergamot oil
½ teaspoon ground cinnamon	2 teaspoons brandy

Mix well before returning to the jar for 2 further weeks to season. Then transfer to potpourri jars.

A Sweet-jar Recipe

½ pound coarse salt
¼ pound saltpeter and kitchen salt
6 baskets rose petals
24 bay leaves, chopped
1 handful myrtle leaves

6 handfuls lavender flowers
1 handful orange
  or syringa blossoms
1 handful violet flowers
1 handful clove carnation flowers

Mix well in a jar every day for a week, and then add:

½ ounce powdered cloves
4 ounces powdered orris root
½ ounce powdered cinnamon
2 nutmegs, ground

An Eighteenth-century Perfume to Mix with Potpourris

4 grains
  (something less than ⅛ teaspoon)
  musk oil or tincture
2 teaspoons ground allspice
2 teaspoons ground cloves

2 teaspoons gum benzoin
80 drops cassia oil
6 drops rose otto (use rose oil)
150 drops bergamot oil
150 drops lavender oil

Mix well with any dried petals you have handy.

Perfume Extracts

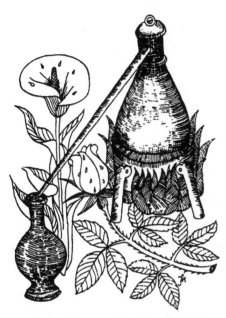

There are three basic methods of extracting the fragrant essential oils from flowers and herbs: 1) distilling in water (the most refined way); 2) steeping in oil, or maceration; and 3) distilling in alcohol (which yields the crudest results). A fourth method, crushing, or expression, is used for fruit only. Not all essential oils are susceptible to all methods. For instance, roses will yield their essence to all three methods, although the finest and most expensive perfume extract, rose otto (also known as attar of roses), is produced by repeated water distillation. Rosemary, on the other hand, is much more susceptible to alcoholic distillation, although it will yield a little to water. Orange flowers and leaves are susceptible to water distillation and maceration, whereas the peel of the fruit, like that of the lemon and lime, yields another type of oil by expression.

Distillation means simply that you boil the herb in predistilled water or denatured and deodorized alcohol, and pass the steam that rises through either a long pipe or, better still, a water-cooled conduit. The steam, which consists of further distilled water and the volatile essential oil from the plant, condenses on the sides of the pipe or conduit and trickles down into the receiver at the other end.

Hungary Water

This is an example of distillation with alcohol. Hungary water is simply oil of rosemary. Supposedly invented for the queen of Hungary by a hermit to cure her paralysis, it is said to be one of the most potent hair restoratives in the herbal pharmacopoeia.[4] The recipe for this extremely fragrant herbal extract is as follows:

Take 1½ pounds fresh, flowering rosemary tops and steep them in 1 gallon denatured wine alcohol for 4 days. At the end of this time distill and preserve the aromatic distillate in closely stoppered vials.

Easier by far for the amateur parfumier, however, is the process of maceration, or enfleurage, as it is known to the trade. This means simply steeping your herb or flower in oil. This method can be used for any herb or fragrant flower you have growing in your garden.

Enfleurage

Simply soak the fresh petals of the flowers or the leaves of the herb in a high-quality odorless oil contained in a covered jelly jar for several days. Professional parfumiers use refined olive oil, but you can use any odorless vegetable or cosmetic oil. I prefer purified mineral oil, obtainable from a pharmacy. It's colorless and odorless and doesn't turn rancid, which olive oil has a tendency to do. Sprinkle a little salt on the petals as a preservative, too. A few drops of tincture of benzoin should be added later. You can line the jelly jar with cheesecloth first if you wish. This will enable you to strain the petals out after a day or two. Don't let the petals rot or mold, but continue to exchange them for fresh batches every day or so until the oil is well and truly perfumed—usually after 4 or 5 changes. You can add a few drops of tincture of benzoin as a fixative now. Finally, filter your finished product through fine muslin or a filter paper into a closely stoppered opaque or semiopaque ceramic or glass vial. Then use it as a perfume either simply or in a blend, or as a body oil, or mix it with a little alcohol to form a cologne or use it in your sachets. You can even dab it on a lamp bulb to perfume your apartment in winter and remind you of summer when the lamp is on.

---

[4] For details of a simple but effective rosemary hair rinse, see p. 241.

Old-fashioned Spiritous Rose Water

So you can't be bothered with distillation or enfleurage, but would still like to preserve the perfume of your roses? All you need for this recipe is a glass bottle with a wide neck and tight top—again a trusty pickle jar will do wonderfully. Fill it ⅔ full of deodorized, denatured alcohol, and then add freshly gathered rose petals (white are best, says the recipe), carnations, jasmine, or whichever aromatic herb you wish—basil, lemon verbena, rosemary, lavender, until the brim is reached. Close tightly and leave to steep for several months in a cool, dark place without opening. Then filter the resultant liquid and bottle. If you don't have any alcohol, an even simpler method of extracting fragrance from herbs is by using distilled vinegar.

Aromatic Vinegars

These have been used by herbalists for a very long time as astringent lotions and hair rinses. Vinegar is simply a botanically derived fermentation, such as wine or beer, in which most of the alcohol has been worked on by bacteria and transformed into acetic acid, like alcohol an excellent preservative.

Steep 1 ounce *dried* aromatic herbs—lavender, rosemary, orris, rosebuds, camomile—whichever you choose, singly or in combination, in 1 pint distilled vinegar for 2 to 3 weeks. Then filter and use diluted with water as an astringent skin lotion or a stimulating and deep-cleansing hair rinse.

Before leaving the subject of do-it-yourself perfume extracts, here is a classic example of perhaps one of the most deliciously fragrant homemade perfume blends yet devised. It went under a variety of different names. The most well known was royal essence.

Royal Essence

25 parts ambergris oil or tincture

12 parts musk oil or tincture

5 parts civet oil or tincture

2 parts rose oil

3 parts cinnamon oil

2 parts oil of rhodium

2 parts neroli oil

(Artificial approximations or blends may be used for the musk, civet, ambergris, and neroli just as effectively, provided they are good ones.) Combine simply as a perfume oil, or mix with deodorized alcohol to the desired strength to form a cologne. Add distilled water to the cologne to make a toilet water.

Incenses

Potpourris and sachets are not, of course, the only means of perfuming or freshening your home. Essential oils may be sped on their way into the atmosphere by the application of heat. We have already mentioned the relatively new and highly effective device of using a dot of essential oil placed on a hot lamp bulb or radiator. The old way of accomplishing the same result was with incense. Incense has always been inextricably linked with religion and magic, and was first used by man as a means of appeasing the gods and spirits. People would light the fires on which they burned sacrificial meats and foods with sweet-smelling woods like bay, laurel, and sandal. The aromatic smoke that drifted up would obviously please the gods in their celestial abodes as much as the food. When sacrifice fell into abeyance, the practice of praying over perfumed smoke remained. Resins such as frankincense and galbanum and storax were blended with other exotic ingredients like the now-unavailable onycha, to form the priestly incenses burned in the inner sanctuaries of temples. The use of incense acquired an occult mystique when Babylonian astrology infiltrated European paganism during the first 400 years after Christ. The Neoplatonists, groups of pagans who practiced a composite religion made up of doctrines and deities drawn from the ancient Egyptians, Greeks,

Romans, and Babylonians, passed their arcane beliefs on to unorthodox Christian sects known as the Gnostics, who in turn were drawn on by Arabian occult philosophers. These magi, who called themselves Sabians, laid special stress on the use of astrological prayers, sacrifices, and suffumigations, and the works of the greatest among them, Thebit ben Corat, were the source books for all later medieval grimoires, books of sorcery and necromancy used by wizards to conjure up demons and ghosts. In the Western religions that survive today, only the Roman Catholic, High Anglican, and Greek Orthodox churches now use incense. It is, however, still used extensively in the rites of the two great religions of the East, Buddhism and Hinduism.

Although incense burning was tossed out as so much superstition by the Protestant churches, it still held its own in a minor way as a means of perfuming the home. Many of the old manorial still-room books of the eighteenth and nineteenth centuries list incense recipes, as do the printed "housewife's companion" booklets of Victorian times. Most of the recipes are unnecessarily complicated. As with sachets and potpourris, once you understand the principles of incense blending you can go ahead and cook up your own quite satisfactorily.

HOW TO MAKE INCENSE

There are three types of ingredients that go into the composition of self-burning household incense cones or sticks: 1) the aromatic substance; 2) a chemical to keep it burning; and 3) a bonding agent to hold it all together.

1. The Aromatic Substance

The aromatic substance is generally an herb, wood, resin, or simply odorless powdered wood scented with an essential oil. Not all fragrant herbs smell good when you burn them. Try incinerating a little spearmint, for example, and see how the fetid moke differs from, say, the lovely aroma of burned thyme or bay leaves.

Useful Incense Herbs, Woods, and Spices

Allspice berries (spicy-smelling)

Balm of Gilead buds (delicious and heady aroma)

Bay leaves (mellow)

Birch bark (piney)

Calamus root (sweet, fruity)

Cascarilla bark (gives a good "musk" smell when burned)

Cassia bark (cinnamonlike)

Cedarwood leaves and shavings (mellow)

Cinnamon bark (warm and spicy, like the flavor)

Cloves (warm and spicy, like the flavor)

Cubeb berries (spicy)

Cypress leaves and shavings (bittersweet)

Deer's tongue leaves (delicious and heady)

Dittany of Crete leaves (herby)

Eucalyptus leaves (like camphor)

False winter's bark (*Cinnamodendron corticosum*; like cinnamon)

Fir needles (sweet and piney)

Juniper leaves and shavings (piney)

Lavender flowers (fabulous)

Life everlasting leaves (herby)

Lignum aloes (*Aquilaria agallocha*; woodsy)

Marjoram leaves (herby)

Myrrh wood (may be used in place of gum myrrh)

Myrtle leaves (eucalyptuslike)

Orris root (violetlike; I am not as keen on orris as an incense as many old recipes are)

Patchouli leaves (fantastic; a major ingredient in Chinese incenses)

Pepperwort herb (a type of dittany; pleasantly woodsy)

Pine needles (piney, obviously; the Chinese burned these to chase evil spirits out of their homes)

Rosemary (delicious; once used as incense in Medieval Europe)

Rose petals (a bit like an autumn bonfire, but some people like them)

Sage leaves (herby)

Sandalwood (again, fantastic; a prime ingredient of most Indian incense)

Sassafras wood (sweet, and very native American)

Sea wormwood (*Artemisia cina*; bitter and pungent)

Southernwood leaves (rather pungent; an old standby for purging kitchen odors, on the principle of one nail driving out another)

Star anise bark (used principally in Japanese incense)

Sumbul root (another excellent substitute for musk; Persian incense used to employ sumbul extensively)

Tansy leaves (sweet and herby)

Thyme leaves (sweet and woodsy)

Tonka beans (vanillalike)
Vetivert (delicious)
Water agrimony flowers (*Bidens tripartita;* smells like cedar)
Winters bark (cinnamonlike smell; useful mainly as a wood base with an essential oil)
Woodruff leaves (very fragrant; vanillalike)
Wormwood leaves (bitter, but interesting)

Any of these herbs and woods may be burned singly or in combination to produce an aromatic smoke. With one exception—balm of Gilead buds—they have to be smoldered to release their fragrance. Balm of Gilead, however, contains a great deal of resin and needs only the gentle application of heat to release its fragrant essential oil.

Useful Incense Gums

The word "gum" used in this context is actually a little inaccurate. What are known in incense making as incense gums and in varnish making and elsewhere as gum resins are simply the resins exuded by certain trees, mostly of the conifer variety. A gum is water-soluble, a resin is not. Hence the use of resins as picture varnishes. Resins and balsams (known as oleo-resins, half essential oil and half resin) burn with a smoky flame and give off their essential oil when heated. Consequently, for best effect they have to be fumed rather than burned on top of a heated metal plate or on a piece of glowing charcoal. Resins are the chief ingredient of the incenses of the Catholic and Orthodox churches, the most widely used being frankincense, with myrrh, benzoin, and galbanum added in lesser amounts, depending on the grade of incense involved. The best grade, often called "high altar" incense, is generally pure frankincense alone.

Here are the resins and balsams which you can use as incense:

Benzoin, gum (very aromatic; there are 2 varieties: Sumatra, sweet and rather like storax; and Siamese, which has a vanillalike fragrance)

Balsam of Peru (sweet-smelling)
Balsam of tolu (sweet-smelling)
Gum bdellium (an inferior type of myrrh; bitter)
Camphor, gum (cold and spicy)

Dragon's-blood resin (*Calamus draco*; sweetly pungent; once used as a red pigment and lacquer)

Frankincense, gum, or olibanum (like lavender; exquisite aroma)

Galbanum, gum (gorgeously bittersweet)

Mastic, gum (a sharp, light aroma)

Myrrh, gum (bitter and mysterious)

Opopanax, gum (dark and bittersweet)

Sandarac, gum (cedarlike)

Storax, gum, or stacte (cloyingly sweet)

Thus, gum (piney)

Lastly, any of your favorite essential oils.

2. The Chemical

If you are using a thurible or a glowing charcoal block to burn your incense, you won't need to add any chemicals to your blend. However, most household incenses and Oriental brands do away with the necessity of thuribles or charcoal by incorporating the same slow-burning chemical additive found in cigarette papers and the fuses of fireworks, potassium nitrate, otherwise known as nitre or saltpeter. The proportion of potassium nitrate (available from the pharmacy) to your other ingredients should be not more than 1 part in 10; otherwise its smell will become overpowering. So if you have mixed up a 2-pound batch of incense, plan on adding up to 3 ounces saltpeter.

With this type of incense you cannot use resins alone, however; they must be combined with at least twice as much aromatic powdered woods, herbs, or charcoal for the saltpeter to work effectively. It doesn't matter how large the proportion of woods and herbs are, as long as the resins do not exceed half their bulk proportionately.

3. The Bonding Agent

If you have included both an essential oil and a resin in your incense blend, you may find that the oil combines with the resin to provide a very gummy bonding agent. Incense cones, or pastilles, may then be modeled and allowed to dry without further complication. However, if the proportion of oil and resin is too low, or if you wish to dip wooden splints and make them into joss sticks and the paste is too thick, you will need to add a bonding agent. In this instance use a vegetable gum of some sort. The two most commonly employed are acacia gum, generally known as gum arabic, and gum tragacanth, the sap of the *Astragalus gummifer* shrub. Both are available from art-supply stores, pharmacies, and many herb mail-order companies.

Simply add enough gum to make the incense into a paste thin enough to adhere to the splints. If the gum comes in solid form, add boiling water (2 parts water to 1 part gum) and leave to soak for several hours. When the powder has well and truly dissolved, add enough gum to your incense to make it into a paste. Then dip the splints in it, and stick them in a polystyrene block or a lump of modeling clay to dry. If you make several types of joss stick, try adding a few drops of various colored inks or food dyes to each batch of incense mix also to distinguish them from one another.

ANCIENT INCENSE RECIPES

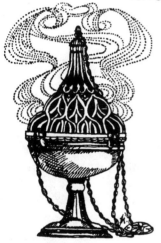

BYZANTINE THURIBLE

About the most ancient incense recipe we have on hand is that used by the priests of old Egypt in their temples. There are various papyrus accounts of the components of *kyphi*, as the incense was called. Most of them, though consistent with one another up to a certain point, omit to mention proportions. Only one does this: the recipe given by Dioscorides himself, and translated in 1655 by John Goodyer. Here they all are for comparison.

Kyphi

Papyrus Recipe I

Resin
Wine
Galangal root
Juniper berries
Aromatic rush root

Asphaltum (probably a
  mistranslation of *Aspalathus*,
  or broom)
Mastic gum
Myrrh gum
Grapes
Honey

Papyrus Recipe II

Honey	Calamus
Wine	Asphaltum (broom plant)
Raisins	Thyron (frankincense)
Sweet rush	Dock
Resins (probably pine resin)	Both kinds of arceuthids
Myrrh	(the lesser and the
Frankincense	greater juniper)
Seselis (probably a	Cardamoms
variety of saxifrage)	Orris root

One has to remember that kyphi was used not only as an incense but as a medicine too, hence the presence of the wine, honey, and raisins. These substances also make it seem highly unlikely that the kyphi was always burned, being either fumed on top of hot metal or poured on top of a sacrificial offering rather as one would add a sauce to a dish to give it extra flavor.

Dioscorides' Recipe for Kyphi

"Cyphi is the composition of a perfume, wellcome to ye Gods: The Priests in Egypt doe use it abundantly. It is mixt also with Antidots, and it is given to the Asthmaticall in drinkes. There are many waies of the making of it carryed about, in which this also is: Take one half a sextarium [½ pint] of Cyperus [*Cyperus odoratus*, sweet sedge root], of full Juniper berries as much, of plum raisins of the Sun stoned twelve poundes; Resinae repurgatae [refined rosin] 5 lb., of Calamus Aromaticus [calamus root], of Aspalathus [*Genista acanthoclada*, broom plant], and of Iuncus odoratus [lemon grass], of each a pounde, of Myrrh twelve dragms [1½ ounces], of old wine nine sextarios [9 pints] of Hony twoe lb. Having taken out the stones of the raisins, pound the Raisins, and worke them together with wine and Myrrh, and pounding and sifting the other thinges mix them with these, and let them drinck up the liquor one day. Afterward seething the Hony, till it comme to a glutinous consistence, mix the Rosin being melted carefully with it, and then having pounded all the other thinges diligently together, put them up into a vas fictile [earthenware pot]."

Moses' Temple Incense

"And the Lord said unto Moses, Take unto thee sweet spices, stacte, and onycha, and galbanum; these sweet spices with pure frankincense: of each shall there be a like weight: And thou shalt make it a perfume, a confection after the art of the apothecary, tempered together, pure and holy." (Exodus 30: 34–35)

Ancient Roman Incenses

The Romans burned these to accompany bloodless sacrifices, that is, offerings made to the gods comprising fruit, corn, loaves, wine, and so on.

I. Olive wood, Bay leaves, Pitchwood (pine), Savine wood.

II. Frankincense, Myrrh, Crocus (saffron), Costum (*Saussurea lappa*).

A Seventeenth-century Incense

Sir Kenelm Digby was a colorful philosopher-scientist of the seventeenth century. Colorful because he also happened to be an able politician, soldier, doctor, astrologer, and herbalist—in fact, practically everything. He was friendly with kings Charles I and II, Bacon, Galileo, Descartes, and Cromwell. His delightful books on herbalism, alchemy, and allied subjects are a direct consequence of the experiments he performed in the laboratory of his grand house in Covent Garden. In Digby's *Receipts in Physick and Chirurgery* (1668) we come across the following rudimentary incense formula:

> Take half a pound of Damask Rosebuds [the whites cut off], Benjamin [benzoin] three ounces beaten to powder, half a quarter of an ounce of Musk, and as much of Ambergris, the like of Civet. [Those three magical ingredients again!] Beat all these together in a stone Morter. Then put in an ounce of Sugar, and make it up in Cakes, and dry them in the Sun, or by the fire.

Two Victorian Household Incenses

The Victorians added saltpeter to their incenses to make them more combustible:

I.

4 ounces gum benzoin
½ ounce cascarilla bark
  (*Croton eleutheria*)
3 drams (3 teaspoons) saltpeter
3 drams (3 teaspoons) gum arabic

1 dram (1 teaspoon) gum myrrh
25 drops oil of nutmeg
25 drops oil of cloves
7 ounces charcoal

Powder and mix the ingredients well before adding enough cold water to form a paste suitable to form cones or pastilles or dip splints in. Allow to dry thoroughly before attempting to use.

II.

3 ounces white sandalwood
4 ounces gum storax
3 ounces gum benzoin
6 ounces gum frankincense
6 ounces cascarilla bark
1 teaspoon ambergris (oil
  or tincture)
2 teaspoons balsam of Peru
1½ ounces gum myrrh
1½ ounces saltpeter

20 drops cinnamon (or cassia) oil
½ teaspoon oil of cloves
30 to 60 drops rose otto (use
  rose oil)
1½ teaspoons lavender oil
1½ ounces balsam of tolu
½ ounce gum camphor
2 ounces strong acetic acid
  (vinegar)
3 pounds charcoal

Pound each solid ingredient to a fine powder and mix all well together. Add enough mucilage of tragacanth to make a paste suitable for molding cones or dipping splints. Allow to dry thoroughly before using.

The following measurements are proportional, and may be varied in accordance with the quantity of incense required. Also, make sure your ingredients are all finely ground before mixing them.

Chinese Incense

2 parts ground allspice
2 parts ground cinnamon or cassia
3 parts patchouli leaves
1 part gum myrrh
½ part saltpeter
A few drops ylang ylang or galangal oil
Gum arabic or tragacanth, diluted as required

Tibetan Incense

2 parts white sandalwood
2 parts ground cinnamon or cassia
3 parts powdered cypress, juniper, or cedar leaves or
  wood
1 part gum benzoin
½ part saltpeter
A few drops musk oil
Gum arabic or tragacanth, diluted as required

Japanese Incense

7 parts star anise bark
1 part ground cassia
½ part saltpeter
A few drops almond or cherry blossom oil
Gum arabic or tragacanth, diluted as required

Indian Incense

7 parts white sandalwood
1 part ground cinnamon or cassia
½ part saltpeter
A few drops nutmeg oil
Gum arabic or tragacanth, diluted as required

222 / MASTERING HERBALISM

Persian Incense

4 parts white sandalwood
3 parts ground sumbul root
1 part gum frankincense
½ part saltpeter
A few drops rose or jasmine oil
Gum arabic or tragacanth, diluted as required

Egyptian Incense

7 parts cedarwood
1 part gum myrrh
½ part saltpeter
A few drops juniper oil
A few drops lemon, bergamot, or citronella oil
Gum arabic or tragacanth, diluted as required

Mix ingredients into a well-blended paste and model it into cones or dip splints of wood in it. Allow to dry well before using.

A Simple Sandalwood Incense

10 ounces powdered sandalwood
1 pound powdered gum benzoin
3 pounds crushed charcoal (obtain this from a pharmacy or use the willow charcoal obtainable from art-supply stores)
5½ ounces balsam of tolu
7 ounces saltpeter
Gum arabic as required

Mix ingredients into a well-blended paste and model it into cones or dip splints of wood in it. Allow to dry well before using.

Roman Catholic Liturgical Incense

10 parts gum frankincense (olibanum)
4 parts gum benzoin (benjamin)
1 part gum storax (stacte)

Pulverize and mix well.

HOW TO BURN NONIGNITING INCENSES

If you don't want to use saltpeter, you will need to fume your incense on a charcoal block. Ideally this should be set in a fireproof incense burner. If you don't own one, never mind. Any handy-sized bowl or ashtray filled with an inch or two of sand will do the job as effectively. Some people insert a ceramic tile under the bowl as an extra precaution to prevent scorching the tabletop. Just place your charcoal block (obtainable from most religious supply stores and some mail-order companies) in the bowl on top of the sand, apply a match, and stand back. When the block has finished fizzing sprinkle a few grains of your incense on it. Then sit back and enjoy, meditate, or read a book.

ASTROLOGICAL INCENSE

According to Francis Barrett, a nineteenth-century London sorcerer who practiced what he preached to the extent of running a bona fide college of wizardry in Marylebone High Street (two steps away from Baker Street), these are the incenses which would invoke the influences of the planets and the signs of the zodiac. If astrology intrigues you, these are the fragrances traditionally ascribed to the birth signs; they can be blended into incenses for yourself and your friends.

Zodiacal Birth-sign Perfumes

♈ Aries	(March 21–April 19):	myrrh
♉ Taurus	(April 20–May 20):	pepperwort (*Lepidium latifolium*)
♊ Gemini	(May 21–June 21):	mastic
♋ Cancer	(June 22–July 22):	camphor
♌ Leo	(July 23–August 22):	frankincense

♍ Virgo	(August 23–September 22):	sandalwood
♎ Libra	(September 23–October 22):	galbanum
♏ Scorpio	(October 23–November 21):	opopanax
♐ Sagittarius	(November 22–December 21):	aloes *(Aquilaria agallocha)*
♑ Capricorn	(December 22–January 19):	benzoin
♒ Aquarius	(January 20–February 18):	euphorbium
♓ Pisces	(February 19–March 20):	red storax

To make a really personalized incense for yourself or for someone you know, add one of the following perfumes:

Planetary Perfumes for the Days of the Week

♄ Saturn	(Saturday):	pepperwort or any root
♃ Jupiter	(Thursday):	nutmeg or any fruit
♂ Mars	(Tuesday):	lignum aloes or any wood
☉ Sun	(Sunday):	mastic or any gum
♀ Venus	(Friday):	saffron or any flower
☿ Mercury	(Wednesday):	cinnamon or any paring or peel
☽ Moon	(Monday):	myrtle or any leaf

Simply combine the birth-sign perfume with that of the day of the week on which the person was born. For instance, if you were born on Friday, March 1, use storax and saffron or any floral essential oils as your dominant perfumes.

Aromatic Candles

You can also make the type of fragrant candle so frequently seen in gift shops for yourself with very little trouble, and using your own favorite essential oils into the bargain. Simply melt a little candle wax in a used coffee can or old saucepan and add a few drops of the essential oil of your choice. Mix thoroughly. Fasten a paper clip to the wick of a regular store-bought candle and suspend it by this over another empty can. Then pour the scented wax over it. Do this several times until the candle has received a good coating of wax. Color pigments may be added to the wax to tint it if desired. Attractive scented astrological candles can also be made in this way, using the perfume categories just mentioned and the following traditional color scheme:

Zodiacal Birth-sign Colors

Aries:	♈	scarlet
Taurus:	♉	red-orange
Gemini:	♊	orange
Cancer:	♋	gold
Leo:	♌	yellow
Virgo:	♍	chartreuse
Libra:	♎	green
Scorpio:	♏	blue-green
Sagittarius:	♐	blue
Capricorn:	♑	blue-black
Aquarius:	♒	violet
Pisces:	♓	magenta

Herbal Smoking Mixtures

While we're on the subject of suffumigations, here is a run-down of herbs you can use as tobacco substitutes:

Basic Smoking Herbs

Bearberry leaves (*Uva-ursi*)
Buckbean leaves (*Menyanthes trifoliata*)
Chervil leaves (*Choerophyllum sativum*)

Coltsfoot leaves (*Tussilago farfara*)
Corn silk (*Stigmeta maidis*)
Dittany leaves (*Cunila mariana*)
Eyebright leaves (*Euphrasia officinalis*)
Life everlasting leaves (*Antennaria dioica*)
Marjoram leaves (*Origanum marjorana*)
Mullein leaves (*Verbascum thapsus*; said to give relief from asthma)
Raspberry leaves (*Rubus strigosus*)
Rosemary leaves (*Rosmarinus officinalis*; mixed with coltsfoot, said to give relief from asthma)
Sage leaves (*Salvia officinalis*; said to give relief from asthma)
Wood betony leaves (*Betonica officinalis*)
Yerba santa (*Eriodictyon californicum*)

Aromatic Smoking Herbs

Also try adding any of these herbs and spices to your herbal tobacco to give it added aroma:

Allspice berries (spicy aroma)
Cascarilla bark (musky)
Cubeb berries (spicy aroma)
Deer's tongue leaves (vanilla aroma)
Eucalyptus leave (menthol aroma)
Lavender flowers (very fragrant)
Licorice root (sweet)
Melilot flowers (vanilla aroma)
Sassafras bark (sweet)
Thyme leaves (incenselike)
Tonka beans (vanilla aroma)
Woodruff leaves (vanilla aroma)

British Herbal Tobacco

This is a pleasant tasting and aromatic smoking mixture which I can heartily recommend to anyone anxious to find a less noxious substitute for tobacco. It can be smoked in a pipe or rolled into cigarettes. Pipe smoking, however, precludes the direct (and harmful) inhalation of saltpeter from the cigarette paper.

16 parts dried coltsfoot leaves	2 parts dried rosemary leaves
8 parts eyebright leaves	1½ parts dried thyme
(*Euphrasia officinalis*)	1 part dried lavender flowers
8 parts buckbean leaves	1 part rose petals (optional)
4 parts wood betony leaves	1 part camomile flowers (optional)

Although they do form part of the recipe, I usually omit the rose and camomile as I find they detract from rather than add to the flavor.

The herbs should be rubbed to a coarse powder through the fingers or the wide mesh of a sieve. Make sure they get a good mixing too. If you prefer a milder blend, increase the proportion of coltsfoot leaves. Any of the aromatic smoking herbs can, of course also be incorporated to give your blend extra distinction.

Intoxicating Smoking Herbs

Finally, here is a list of some of the common herbs that are being used today to give herbal tobaccos that something extra. Unlike cannabis, all these herbs are legally obtainable (as of the time of writing), but some of them at least could be harmful taken to excess. As with all powerful herbs and spices, any good thing can be overdone.

Boldo leaves (rather harsh on the throat)
Broom tops (be careful with these; they can be dangerous)
Catnip leaves
Damiana leaves
Ginseng leaves
Hydrocotyle asiatica minor (stimulant in small doses, narcotic in large)
Lobelia leaves (herbalists use these in asthma preparations; I wouldn't recommend them because, like broom, they can be dangerous)
Passionflower leaves
Poppyheads and leaves (if they're white poppies, then they are opium, and very illegal; however, legal red poppies also have a mild effect)
Wild lettuce juice (also known as lettuce opium; need I say more?)
Yarrow leaves

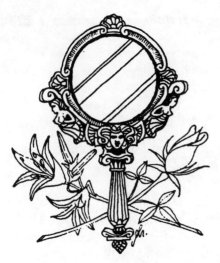

HERBAL BEAUTY SECRETS

Centuries before inorganic chemistry took over in the field of cosmetics, herbs played a large part in the composition of beauty preparations. Most of the great beauties and courtesans of the past possessed, or were thought to possess, their own pet beauty secrets which partially accounted for their grand success in *les choses d'amour*. Many of these secrets did, in fact, involve herbs and spices. Interestingly enough, several large cosmetic companies are now adding herbal preparations to their lists of shampoos and deodorants. It seems that the wheel has turned full cycle. One feels that Madame de Lenclos, Molière's beautiful confidante, could only have approved the current trend. She always knew best when it came to matters of love and beauty, or so her biographers say. The secret of her enduring success—85 years of it—was said to have lain in the herbal baths she took. We are indeed lucky to still possess her formula, which is simple enough:

Ninon de Lenclos's Bath Sachet

Take equal parts of lavender flowers, rosemary, spearmint, comfrey roots, and thyme and mix them loosely in a muslin bag. Allow them to steep at least 10 minutes in a little boiling-hot water before adding the remainder of the bath water. Then step in and "think virtuous thoughts."

Marie Antoinette's Bath Sachet

That other renowned but ill-fated French beauty, Marie Antoinette, also had an herbal bath recipe, in which, it was whispered, lay the secret of her beauty, if not her long life:

> 1 part wild thyme *(Thymus serpyllum)*
> 1 part marjoram
> 1 part coarse salt

A trifle rustic, maybe, but then she did enjoy dressing up as a shepherdess.

HERBAL BATHS IN GENERAL

There is really nothing so revolutionary or special about Madame de Lenclos's bath habits. These were the old days, before sophisticated bath salts and "gelées" were invented, and people had used herbs to scent their bath water since Roman times. The herbs, however, did carry an added bonus which most of today's commercial bath salts lack: their medicinal properties. Nature has provided us with three natural means of access to our bloodstream: through our stomach, through our lungs, and through our skin. When we soak ourselves in herbal baths we are using the latter. Of course, all and any baths are good for us, herbal or not: for one thing, they serve to clean out all our pores, tiny vents that pepper the surface of our skins and excrete toxic waste matter from our bodies; and for another, they obviously relax and soothe sore muscles and joints.

Any of your regular herbal sachets can be used as a bath sachet too. However, if you want to make up a sachet specially for the bath, try adding an equal amount of borax crystals to the herbs to soften the water. Vetivert makes one of the best bath-sachet fixatives, so add some of that too. If you do this, you will be able to re-use the sachet several times. But, remember that a bath sachet can contain active, that is, medicinally potent, as well as inactive and merely fragrant, herbs. Consult Chapter 1 for the type of herb you require, soothing or stimulant, but steer clear of those like rue, which can have allergenic side effects.

One last tip before you wallow: you will get best results from a sachet if you knead and squeeze it first under the hot tap before allowing it to steep in your bath. Also, soak yourself for at least 10 minutes to give the herbs enough time to take effect.

Common Bath Sachet Ingredients

Balm leaves (stimulating)
Basil leaves (stimulating)
Bay leaves (stimulating)
Camomile (common) flowers (stimulating)
Catnip leaves (relaxing)
Comfrey leaves and roots (soothing to the skin)
Elder flowers (relaxing)
Fennel seeds and leaves (stimulating)
German camomile (relaxing)
Hop flowers (relaxing)
Horse chestnut bark (relaxing)
Jasmine flowers (relaxing)
Lavender flowers (stimulating)
Lemon peel (stimulating)
Lemon verbena (stimulating in a bath)
Linden flowers (relaxing)
Lovage leaves (stimulating)

Marigold petals (stimulating)
Meadowsweet flowers (stimulating)
Melilot flowers (soothing to the skin)
Oatmeal (for itchy skin)
Orange leaves and flowers (stimulating)
Pennyroyal leaves (stimulating)
Peppermint leaves (stimulating)
Pine needles (stimulating)
Rosebuds (stimulating)
Rosemary leaves (stimulating)
Sage leaves (stimulating)
Sandalwood, white (stimulating)
Skullcap leaves (relaxing)
Spearmint leaves (stimulating)
Thyme (stimulating)
Valerian root (relaxing)
Vetivert (stimulating)
Yarrow flowers (stimulating)

If you don't have the herbs, but would like to get the general effect of their perfume, then use just the essential oils in the following manner:

Homemade Bath Salts

5 ounces bicarbonate of soda
5 ounces tartaric acid
3 ounces powdered orris root
A few drops of your favorite essential oils

Pound and mix all the ingredients well and keep them in a decorative closed jar. Dissolve a handful of salts in the bath water before stepping in.

Simple Bath Salts

If you want to try a simplified version of the above recipe, omit the tartaric acid and orris and use only the bicarbonate of soda and your essential oils. Like borax, the soda neutralizes the acids secreted by your pores and gives a marvelous soft quality to the water that is relaxing and refreshing.

The Herbal Steam Bath

Steam baths have long been recognized as a fine way of opening up the pores and cleansing the body and skin of toxic impurities. Many health resorts are now adding fresh herbs to their saunas and facials, too. As we have seen, herbs yield their essential oils to heat, and it is these oils that act directly on the skin as bracers and tonics. Most of the herbs employed for steam saunas and facials are therefore those known to be rich in fragrant essential oils. Here are some of the easily obtainable ones you can use:

For All Skin

Basil leaves	Eucalyptus leaves	Spearmint leaves
Camomile flowers	Linden flowers	Thyme leaves
Cloves	Peppermint leaves	Verbena leaves

Astringents for Oily Skin

Lavender flowers	Orange leaves, peel,	Rosemary leaves
Lemon grass	and flowers	Sage leaves
Lemon leaves,	Rosebuds	Yarrow flowers
peel, and flowers		

Emollients for Dry Skin

Clover tops	Melilot flowers
Elder flowers	Primrose flowers

Infuse a handful of the herbs of your choice, loose or in sachet form, in a large bowl of boiling water. Place a towel over your head and hold your face over the bowl for 10 to 15 minutes, inhaling deeply. Finally, rinse your face with cold water to close the pores once more. Try it and you will see how refreshing it is.

HERBAL SKIN CLEANSERS

Opening the pores is sometimes only half the battle; often stronger methods are required to draw out unsightly blackheads. Probably two of the most useful skin cleansers ever known to herbalists are almonds and oatmeal. Almonds have been used since biblical times as a food and cosmetic. Almond oil is a commonplace in today's skin care and cosmetics, but the raw almond itself can be just as useful. Both oatmeal and almond meal possess an extraordinary capacity for drawing out the impurities from clogged pores (which is all that blackheads are), and their astringent properties then serve to reduce the pores to a reasonable size once more.

Almond Face Pack

Simply mix a little almond meal (obtainable at a grocery or pharmacy) with water to form a paste, and spread this liberally on your face or other affected areas. Allow the mask plenty of time to dry good and hard before gently rinsing off.

A Seventeenth-century Almond "Paste for ye Hands"

(After making this you may find it difficult to resist eating it rather than working it into ye Hands.)

"Take a pound of Sun raysens, store and take a pound of bitter Almonds, blanch ym and beat ym in stone mortar, with a glass of sack (Madeira or Sherry) take ye peel of one Lemond, boyle it tender; take a quart of milk, and a pint of Ale, and make therewith a Possett (a hot milk drink curdled with ale or wine); take all ye

Curd and putt it to ye Almonds: nb putt in ye Rayson: Beat all till they come to a fine Past, and putt in a pott, and keep it for ye use."

Oatmeal Face Pack

Mix a little ground oatmeal with buttermilk or the white of an egg, and spread it liberally on your face as above. Again, allow at least 20 minutes for the mask to dry and draw before rinsing off. Follow up with an herbal steam facial for extra effect.

SIMPLE BOTANICAL BALMS AND LOTIONS

Did you know that just about any fresh fruit can be used as a cosmetic? For instance:

AVOCADOS. Excellent for lubricating and moisturizing dry skins.

BANANAS. Likewise superb lubricants.

CUCUMBERS. Probably the most widely used item of all in herbal cosmetics. Invaluable for whitening and cleansing, toning up, and generally smoothing away all wrinkles and blemishes. Long valued for their legendary "cooling" properties, they remain, together with elder flowers, the naturalist beautician's panacea.

ORANGES AND LEMON. All citrus fruits are astringent and, like cucumber, tighten the skin and thereby remove wrinkles. In addition to this, lemon also possesses oxidizing properties, and has therefore had a long history as a mild, natural skin and hair bleach.

RASPBERRIES AND STRAWBERRIES. Fragrant and astringent properties make these useful additives to any face packs or masks.

PEACHES AND NECTARINES. Pulpy fruit of any type may be puréed with milk and used as a cleansing skin refresher.

Avocado or Banana Skin Cleanser

Blend a half-ripened banana or avocado with a beaten egg yolk and ½ cup milk and apply gently to the face. Leave for 5 minutes and then rinse off.

Simple Cucumber Lotion

For dried, chapped hands, grate ½ cucumber and strain juice into a blender. Mix in enough olive oil to make a thick lotion. Rub well into the skin.

Cucumber and Quince Blossom Lotion

An old-time facial conditioner:

4 quarts fresh quince blossoms, rose petals, or primrose flowers
2 large cucumbers, grated

Cover the blossoms with water and simmer for 1 hour. Add the cucumber and continue to boil for 5 minutes more. Strain and cool. Leave on the face for at least 10 minutes before washing off.

Cucumber and Elder Flower Lotion

For use on rough or chapped skin.
Peel and slice 1 or 2 large cucumbers and cook them slowly in a double boiler until soft. Filter all the juice out through cheesecloth or thin muslin, and add ¼ its volume of rectified spirits of wine (brandy) or whiskey, and ⅓ its volume of elder flower water. Shake well and bottle for use.

Cucumber and Rose Water Lotion

For rough, dried skin and sunburn.
Mix equal quantities cucumber juice, rose water (obtainable from the pharmacy), and glycerine. Apply liberally where needed.

Cucumber and Witch Hazel Lotion

Witch hazel (*Hamamelis virginiana*) is a shrub which yields an astringent extract from its fresh leaves and young twigs that is still highly prized by the cosmetics industry. Rather than distilling it for yourself, it is of course far simpler to buy the prepared witch hazel extract from a pharmacist. That goes for your rose water too.
This particular lotion should be used as a moisturizer for oily skins.

6 ounces cucumber juice
3 ounces rose water
3 ounces witch hazel

Cucumber Egg Mask

The whites of eggs also possess the property of tightening the skin and thus removing, at least temporarily, unsightly pouches and wrinkles. Combining them with the astringent properties of cucumber, an easy and natural face mask for oily or regular skins can be whipped up at a moment's notice. Use the white of 1 egg beaten stiff, blended with 4 tablespoons cucumber juice. Give the mask about ¼ hour to dry before rinsing off. Follow up with an astringent lotion or simply a cold rinse.

Elder Flower Lotion

Said by herbalists to be effective for treating any skin conditions. Mrs. Grieve called it "healing, cooling and soothing." Indeed, elder flowers, like cucumber, are a standby in cosmetic herbalism, and crop up again and again in this context in the old herbals and still-room books.

Take 2½ drachms (teaspoons) dried elder flowers and pour over them 1 quart boiling water. Cover and leave them to steep for 1 hour before straining and using.

Elder Ointment

This has long been a highly respected ointment among herbalists for its soothing and softening effect on the skin. Mrs. Grieve even recommends it for any kind of tumors, swelling, or wound. Take of the following fresh herbs:

8 ounces elder leaves
4 ounces plantain leaves
2 ounces ground ivy (*Glechoma hederacea*)
4 ounces wormwood

Chop them finely and boil them in 4 pounds of lard (or Vaseline, oil, or other fatty medium) in an oven or over a slow flame. When the leaves become crisp strain them out of the ointment before reserving it for future use.

Lemon Hand Lotion

For gentle cleansing and removal of stains from the hands:

> 1 ounce strained lemon juice
> 3 ounces rose water
> 1 ounce glycerine

Mix ingredients and apply liberally as often as needed.

Marsh-mallow Ointment

Another famous emollient ointment among herbalists:

Old Recipe

> 2 ounces slippery elm bark powder (*Ulmus fulva*)
> 3 ounces marsh-mallow leaves
> 3 pints water
> 3 ounces beeswax
> 16 ounces clarified lard
> A few drops of your favorite aromatic essential oil

Boil the slippery elm and marsh mallow in 3 pints water for 15 minutes. Strain the juice and continue to boil it down to ½ pint. Melt the wax and lard together and add the herbal extract and essential oil while they are still warm (not hot). Mix thoroughly and store in a cool place.

New Recipe

Instead of using lard and beeswax, glycerine and stearic acid may be substituted in the following manner:

> 4 fluid drams (4 teaspoons) glycerine
> 4 ounces stearic acid
> ½ ounce sodium carbonate
> 16 fluid ounces (2 cups) water
> 20 fluid ounces (2½ cups) herbal extract
> Selected essential oils

Mix the glycerine, stearic acid, and sodium carbonate in a large enamel or Pyrex pan and heat gently until the solution clears and the effervescence ceases. Simmer for 60 minutes, topping up with water from time to time to maintain a constant level. Remove from the heat and beat in the herbal extract and selected essential oils.

This recipe may also be used to compose any type of ointment from a prepared herbal extract, for instance, elder flower, cucumber, primrose, or rosemary.

Herbal Creams

A completely oil-free herbal cream may be made as follows. The recipe calls for quince seeds, seeds rich in natural mucilage and therefore useful in the composition of any type of herbal ointment or emollient rub.

1 ounce quince seeds	⅔ teaspoon borax
4 ounces glycerine	2 ounces water
7 cups herbal essence	4 ounces purified alcohol

Steep the quince seeds in the glycerine and herbal essence for 12 hours, stirring frequently. Strain out the seeds, and into the liquid blend the borax dissolved in the water, and lastly the alcohol as a preservative.

Easy Herbal Cream Base

Simpler still for those lacking the time or inclination to mess with quince seeds and glycerine is the following modern cosmetic formula for a basic herbal cream:

4 ounces any of the following oils:

Almond	Cottonseed	Poppy seed
Apricot kernel	Cucumber	Safflower
Avocado	Lanolin	Sesame
Cocoa butter	Olive	Sunflower
Coconut	Peach kernel	Turtle
Corn	Peanut	

1 ounce beeswax (to solidify the cream)
15 minims (¼ teaspoon) tincture of benzoin
1 ounce filtered herbal extract

Melt the oil and beeswax together in a double boiler, then add the tincture of benzoin and herbal essence. Whip them well together, or better still blend in an electric kitchen blender. As it cools it will thicken. Store in a regular cold cream jar.

Rose Ointment

(By any other name, homemade cold cream.)

1½ ounces spermaceti
1½ ounces white wax
9 ounces almond oil
7 fluid ounces rose water
8 minims (drops) rose oil

Melt and mix well the spermaceti, wax, and almond oil. Add the rose water and rose oil; mix well and store for use. (Instead of rose oil, any of your favorite essential oils, such as bergamot or ylang ylang, may be used.)

Sage and Yarrow Skin Lotions

Infusions of sage, parsley, lime flowers, and yarrow leaves have all been used as astringent lotions for refining the pores of oily skins.

Infuse 1 ounce dried herb or herbs in 1 pint boiling water for 15 minutes. Then apply the hot infusion to the face with a clean washcloth repeatedly several times a day. Even acne is said to respond to this treatment.

Herbs for Your Hair

Herbs have been used in hair rinses since very early times. The Egyptians and Greeks employed henna leaves (*Lawsonia alba* and *inermis*) to dye their hair various shades of red and gold, and they used the flowers to compose a massage ointment. Henna dyeing, although popular in the East, was not introduced to Europe until 1890. Today it has largely been replaced by the chemical dyes obtainable at the cosmetics counter, although it is still in the inventory of most herb sellers. Various shades of red and gold are obtained by mixing it with other herbs such as indigo or sage.

COLORED RINSES FOR THE HAIR

Combinations of these three rinses may be used to produce many variations of tone.

Sage or Henna Leaf Rinse

For brunette or auburn shades: Infuse up to ½ ounce sage leaves (brunette), or henna (auburn) in 1 quart boiling water for ½ hour. Cool and strain before using. Again, the strength of color obtained will depend on how much of the herb you infuse.

Camomile Rinse

A fragrant rinse to bring out the highlights of blond hair. Boil 3 tablespoons camomile flowers in 1 pint water for ½ hour. Cool and then strain; use only after shampooing.

The two most widely used herbal hair tonics, on the other hand, are probably nettle leaves and rosemary.

HAIR TONICS

Nettle Hair Tonic

1 ounce nettle leaves (*Urtica dioica*)
1 pint water
Essential oil or cologne of your choice
1 pint white wine vinegar

Simmer the nettles in the water and vinegar for 2 hours in an enamel pan. Leave to cool, and then strain and add a few drops of the cologne or essential oil of your choice before bottling. Shake well and apply to the scalp every other night.

Rosemary Hair Wash

Rosemary, like nettles, has long been thought to stimulate the hair roots to new activity and prevent premature baldness. Mrs. Grieve claims it as one of the best hair washes known. It certainly smells and feels good. Whether it does actually prevent your hair from falling out is difficult to tell. Maybe it does; it's certainly been attested to long enough.

> 1 ounce dried rosemary leaves and tops
> 1 pint water
> 4 teaspoons borax

Infuse the rosemary in the boiling water in a covered nonmetallic container until the liquid has cooled. Strain and add the borax. Use cold as a hair rinse.

Rosemary Hair Oil

To make a fragrant and tonic hair oil suitable for those who suffer from that dry, unmanageable hair, simply mix oils of sweet almond and rosemary together in a ratio of 3 to 1 (3 of almond, one of rosemary).

VINEGAR RINSES

As we have already noted, herbal vinegars were once relied upon extensively as hair rinses and astringent lotions. Today many people are rediscovering their usefulness in these areas, particularly the former. They really do seem to cleanse and add luster to the hair. To make an herb vinegar, simply take 1 ounce of any combination of fragrant herbs of your choice—lavender flowers, rosebuds, rosemary, orris root, vetivert, lemon verbena—and steep them for up to 3 weeks in 1 cup distilled white vinegar. A drop of extra essential oil, balsam of tolu, or tincture of benzoin may also be added for extra zing.

Floral Hair Rinse

1 ounce lavender flowers
1 ounce jasmine flowers
4 ounces rosebuds
2 pints white wine vinegar
½ pint rose water

Mix all the ingredients in a tall jar and allow them to steep for 2 weeks before straining and bottling the vinegar for use.

NATURAL HERBAL SHAMPOO

A mild, natural, soapless shampoo can be concocted from the bark of the soapwort herb *(Saponaria officinalis)*, commonly known as bouncing bet or latherwort.

4 ounces soapwort bark chips
1 pint distilled water
Essential oil of your choice

Simmer the soapwort in the water until the liquid has been reduced by ½. Allow it to cool, then filter and add a few drops of essential oil. Bottle and use as you would regular shampoo. Failing this, did you know that regular kitchen mayonnaise (real) is about the best shampoo you can use? It contains vinegar, egg, and oil, those three all-important cosmetics; the first to cleanse, the second to provide protein, and the third to add luster!

HERBAL TALCUM POWDERS

These are remarkably easy to make and just as good as any you can buy in the pharmacy. All you need is a basic powder, which may consist of regular unscented talcum, starch, cornstarch, or arrowroot, to which you add your finely powdered herbal ingredients and/or essential oils. Use a ratio of 1 part of any of the following herbs to 1 part powder, and as many drops of your favorite essential oil as you like.

Powdered bayberry bark
Powdered calamus root
Powdered camomile flowers
Powdered cassia buds
Powdered cloves
Powdered cypress leaves
Powdered golden seal
Powdered lavender flowers
Powdered lemon peel
Powdered lime peel
Powdered lignum aloes

Powdered lignum rhodium
Powdered marjoram leaves
Powdered orange peel
Powdered orris root
Powdered patchouli leaves
Powdered rosemary leaves and
    flowers
Powdered rose petals
Powdered sandalwood
Powdered slippery elm bark
Powdered violet flowers

Two Traditional Violet-scented Powders

As you will see, the following recipes contain no hint of the actual herb they are supposed to feature except an approximation of its fragrance, which in its natural state is a delicate and fugitive one. This is a common practice in commercial perfumery, especially now that artificial essential oils have largely replaced the natural ones.

1.

6 parts wheat starch
2 parts orris root powder
2 parts lemon oil
1 part bergamot oil
1 part clove oil

2.

8 ounces starch
1½ ounces orris root powder
10 drops lemon oil
5 drops lavender oil
2 drops clove oil

Pound and mix well the starch and powder; then add oils and mix well.

HERBS TO SLIM WITH

A chapter on beauty secrets would surely not be complete without at least some word on that all-important subject, how to become (and stay) sleek and trim. The day may come when what used to be called pulchritude will find itself back in style again, but that day does seem a long, long way off right now.

Each herbalist will, of course, have his or her own pet methods of treating this pressing problem. Nature, alas, has been a trifle unhelpful here. It almost seems as if we were not meant to be slim, for there really do not appear to be that many herbs that will perform the service of banishing those offending pounds overnight without effort. About the best advice herbalists can give is to eat sparingly and healthfully, omitting starches and carbohydrates and concentrating on protein and salads (that much you knew anyway). Take regular exercise, and drink lots of liquids, particularly teas and fruit and vegetable juices. Especially useful are the "diet" teas, such as agrimony and raspberry leaf. Try not to use sugar; use anise or sweet cicely instead.

Only one plant enjoys a wide reputation among herbalists as an obesity combatter. This is the variety of kelp known as bladderwrack (*Fucus vesiculosis*). Its large iodine content is thought to act directly on the thyroid gland and reduce obesity. Whether this is exactly what happens is not known, but it does seem to work for some people. Bladderwrack infusion or decoction tastes particularly disgusting, however, so it is usually administered in capsule or tablet form (obtainable from most herb companies with pharmaceutical licenses).

During the sixteenth century, chickweed (*Stellaria media*) and fennel were also considered herbs that would "swage" you—that is, make you slender. Herbalists seem to have dropped this application nowadays, but here is the fennel recipe for those anxious to try it. A little lemon and anise in it too would surely not go amiss.

For to Make One Slender [1]

"Take fennel and seethe it in water, a very good quantity, and wring out the juice thereof when it is sod, and drink it first and last [presumably on getting up in the morning and before retiring at night], and it shall swage him or her."

[1] From *The Good Housewife's Jewell*, by T. Dawson (1585).

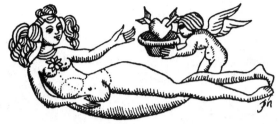

LOVING
HERBS AND APHRODISIACS

AN APHRODISIAC HERB MAY BE defined as one that produces or increases sexual appetite or ability in the user. Therefore it must primarily affect the genital organs and the sex glands. Many herbs have been classified as aphrodisiacs at one time or another merely because they intoxicate and thereby relax inhibitions, thus aiding the user to overcome psychological impotence or frigidity. Cannabis is a good example of this, an herb once known to the Arabs as "increaser of pleasure" on account of this very property. Herbs properly classified as nerve stimulants or tonics have also been labeled aphrodisiacs. Guaiac bark, a popular herbal stimulant, was once known to herbalists as *lignum vitae,* wood of life, for this reason.

Interestingly enough, most of the real aphrodisiacs seem to come from anywhere but Europe. There is no plant indigenous to Europe or the British Isles which can properly be defined as an aphrodisiac. America, the West Indies, the Pacific islands, and the Far East seem to provide the bulk of the real ones, although traditional (but not medicinally valid) loving herbs, such as vervain and southernwood, are indigenous to both Europe and America.

246 / MASTERING HERBALISM

Aphrodisiacs in Antiquity

Nowadays it is widely taken for granted that to perform sexually is as easy and natural as eating or sleeping. However, in the past this was not necessarily the case, especially in primitive conditions. Living in a constant state of stress or fear, or near starvation level in a cave or hut, with little standing between you and the winter's cold with all that it implies—disease, starvation, predatory wild animals—is not really conducive to sexual activity, even though it may be the one entertainment left for those long, dark nights. Birth control is still an alien concept to many people. That babies should be conceived and reared to maturity remains a matter of extreme importance in many societies, especially those based on an agricultural cycle. Where else are the sons to plow the fields and hunt, the daughters to sow the grain and bake the bread, to come from? And equally important to one's own fertility was that of one's crops and livestock, the only food source.

These basic concerns lay behind the development of the ancient fertility religions of Europe, Asia, and North Africa. Their seasonal rituals were supposed to aid the generative processes in man and nature, coax them along, and magnify them at times like midwinter, when the forces of life were in abeyance or hidden underground in the frozen earth. In ancient Egypt the goddess Isis was encouraged to resurrect her dead husband Osiris, who symbolized, for among other things, the corn and the life-bringing waters of the Nile. Next door in Mesopotamia, the lady Ishtar went down to the land of the dead every spring to win back her lover, the nature god Tammuz, from the snares of her sister Ereshkigel; while across the waters of the Mediterranean the Greeks mourned the annual abduction of their corn goddess Persephone by Hades, god of the dead. Many of these fertility cults celebrated their deity's annual disappearance and return with wild dances and erotic rituals, which were in themselves considered helpful in stimulating nature back to life again. Their devotees often seem to have consumed herbal preparations to help them reach a condition of intoxicated religious frenzy. The midnight worshipers of Persephone's son Dionysus chewed ivy leaves to this end. The initiates of Demeter, the Greek earth mother, drank barley brews laced with pennyroyal, and both the Thracians and the Scythians used hemp as a means of attaining collective religious intoxication.

During the first four hundred years A.D. many of these fertility cults found a niche for themselves in imperial Rome. Temples dedicated to Isis flourished side by side with those of Roman, Greek, Asiatic, or Persian deities. Similarly the curious herbal knowledge vested in many of the old fertility religions also ended up in Rome. Caius Petronius, a Roman author of the first century A.D., describes some of the extraordinary measures employed by the priestesses of these cults to cure impotence in his bawdy novel *The Satyricon*. But by Petronius' day many of the cults had lost their solemn religious implications and degenerated into orgiastic secret societies dedicated solely to erotic pursuits, their temples into elaborate brothels. The priestesses themselves were thought of as witches. Chief among the deities served by these sorceresses was the goddess of beauty and love herself, Venus Aphrodite. Our word "aphrodisiac" derives from her name.

Of course, knowledge of aphrodisiac herbs was not solely vested in disreputable sorceresses who peddled love potions, even in the days of Petronius. Dioscorides, who was Petronius' contemporary and a perfectly respectable physician, lists a number of herbs he claims were used as aphrodisiacs, although he also links a number of them to the practices of the "women of Thessaly," that is; to witches. It is interesting to note, however, that he himself does not vouch personally for any of them, but merely records that "it is said that such and such an herb stirs up lust," or words to that effect.

Aphrodisiacs During the Middle Ages

When Christianity finally replaced paganism in Europe, the old fertility cults were branded as lecherous and diabolical, and any type of aphrodisiac came under censure too. The ecclesiastical Council of Trèves of 1310 strictly forbade the use of love potions (among other things) as dangerous and heretical. The action may have been a little heavy-handed, but there was actually a very sound reason behind the rather insubstantial religious one. The unscrupulous and ignorant use of herbs and drugs for aphrodisiac purposes by herb peddlers frequently resulted in terrible and agonizing cases of poisoning.

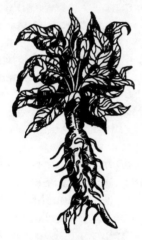

THE MANDRAKE
(*Mandragora officinalis*, or *Atropa mandragora*)

The innocent victim was as often as not secretly given the potion in food in all good faith by an overzealous husband or wife. Such goings-on earned witches and potion peddlers the title *veneficiae*, poisoners, as much as did any arsenical powders for secret murder they might sell. One of the notorious "aphrodisiac" poisons of this type was mandragora, or mandrake root. Another was tincture of cantharides, a violent genital irritant derived from the beetle *Cantharis vesicatoria*. Both Madame de Montespan and Madame de Pompadour, the mistresses of the French kings Louis XIV and Louis XV respectively, dosed their royal lovers secretly with cantharides in an effort to bolster their flagging attentions. It is really quite surprising that both monarchs managed to survive their ladies' solicitude. An eighteenth-century account recorded discreetly in its original French by the author John Davenport in 1869 gives the following rather grotesque description of cantharides poisoning:

> In 1752 we visited a poor man from Organ in Provence afflicted by the most horrible satyriasis one can see or imagine. What happened is this. He had contracted the quartan fever, for which to cure he had consulted a sorceress who made him a potion of an ounce of nettle seeds, two drams of cantharides, a dram and a half of *caboule* and other things, which rendered him so violent in the act of lovemaking that his wife swore to us in God's name that he had mounted her, in two months, eighty-seven times.[1]

The account goes on to describe how the man subsequently died in agony, as is generally the case in severe cantharides poisoning. Obviously not a drug to meddle with!

[1] Author's translation.

Although Europe under Christian influence came to revere chastity as a major virtue in word if not in deed, the East had none of these scruples, and fertility continued to be thought of as a good thing, even under the strict religious rule of Islam. In China and India it occupied a central position in religious and daily life. The *Kama Sutra* of Vatsyayana Malanaga, written during the fourth century A.D., is only one of many popular manuals dealing explicitly with the art of love, a thing unthinkable in Western terms at that time. The Arabs had their own love manuals too, the *Book of Exposition in the Science of Coition* by Jalal al-Din al-Siyuti and the famous *Perfumed Garden* of Sheik Nefzawi, among others. Nefzawi advocated a love potion composed of onion juice, honey, and powdered chickpeas!

Any real knowledge of aphrodisiacs that did filter through to Western herbalists appears to be derived from Dioscorides and these Eastern sources. Western aphrodisiac lore, if one can call it that, seems to have been buried with the ruin of European paganism. The Anglo-Saxon herbals say little or nothing, and Culpeper and Gerard are vague and noncommittal about the whole subject, the former listing only prickly asparagus, dog's mercury, garden mint, white mustard, and onion as herbs suitable for "provoking lust," none of which incidentally have any remote aphrodisiac value from a medicinal point of view. But village wise women still continued to sell their customers potions containing such traditional "aphrodisiacs" as southernwood and vervain. If they did succeed it was probably due more to faith and autosuggestion on the part of the taker than to any recognizable drug resident in the herb. Only when rare East and West Indian herbs and spices became generally available in Europe during the seventeenth and eighteenth centuries did herbal aphrodisiacs become a meaningful concern, albeit still a rather mysterious and naughty one:

"Not only witches, but even naturalists [herbalists] may give potions that incline men and women to lust," tartly commented one disapproving seventeenth-century Scottish lawyer.[2]

---

[2] *Laws and Customs of Scotland in Matters Criminal*, by Sir George Mackenzie (Edinburgh, 1678).

Sexual rejuvenators and love potions have continued to enjoy a brisk market throughout nineteenth- and twentieth-century Europe and America. The "stimulols" and "testogans" of yesterday were, after all, only the descendants of ancient southernwood or vervain brews. Even today there are plenty of herb-derived products around that claim to pep up the sex drive or restore lost potency.

Can aphrodisiacs ever work? Up to a point, yes, if they contain the right drugs to alleviate your condition. There's no point in taking a nerve stimulant if your problem is nervous tension. Like any herbal preparation, they have to be matched to the individual. And in any event, aphrodisiacs are at best only a halfway measure. They cannot conjure up a passion in someone who has none to begin with. The real aphrodisiac turn-on takes place in the mind long before it reaches the sex organs, and is elicited by a groovy love object, not an herb.

Today vitamin E and various types of seeds are widely promoted for their sexually restorative if not necessarily aphrodiasiac properties. Wheat germ and sesame and pumpkin seeds are the chief contenders here. They certainly do appear to be packed full of health-giving vitamins, and although their case as potency-restorers is as yet unproven, they surely cannot do your sex life any harm. Ginseng is another much-promoted aphrodisiac, again unproven, although many, many people follow the example of the ancient Chinese and swear by it. Damiana, another "in" aphrodisiac, is another matter altogether. We shall get to that shortly.

Traditional Aphrodisiacs

DIOSCORIDES' CONTRIBUTION

Orchis

Orchis rubra, O. papilionacea. "Orchus, which some call Cynosorchis, hath leaves about ye stalk strewed upon ye earth, & the bottom of it, like to ye olive being tender, but narrower, &

smooth, & longer, a stalk ye heighth of a span, on which are flowers of a purple hue: roote bulbous, somewhat long, narrow, as of ye Olive, double, the one above, ye other beneath, one full but the other soft & full of wrinkles, but ye root is eaten being sodden like a Bulbus. And of this it is said that if the greater roote is eaten by men, it makes them beget males, & the lesser, being eaten by women, to conceive females. It is further storied that ye women in Thessalia [3] do give to drink with goates milk ye tenderer root to provoke Venerie, & the dry root for ye suppressing, dissolving of Venerie. And that it being drank, ye one is dissolved by the other. It grows in stony, & sandy places."

Saturion (Ophrys sp.)

"Satyrium, but some call it Trifolium ... This one ought to drink in black hard wine for ye Opisthotonon, & use it, if he will lie with a woman. For they say that this also doth stirr up courage in ye conjunction."

Saturion Eruthronion

Erythronium Dens canis Serapiada cordigera or *Morion*. "Satyrium Erythronium, some call it Satyrium Erythraicum (some Melium aquaticum, some Entaticon, or Priapiscus, or Morion or Satyriscus, or testiculum Satyri, ye Romans Molorticulum Veneris) ... It is said that it doth stirr up conjunctions ... It is storied that the root being taken into ye hand doth provoke to Venerie, but much more, being drank with wine."

Gallion (Lady's Bedstraw)

Galium verum. "... ye root doth provoke to conjunction."

Orminon Emeron (Salvia horminum)

"... This also is thought being drank with wine to provoke conjunction."

---

[3] A place notorious for its witches in Dioscorides' day.

So much for Dioscorides. It would be interesting to know if he had ever tried any of these himself. He seems just a little too noncommittal to really carry conviction through.

The following herbs and spices have also been used for centuries all over the world as ingredients of love potions. None of them, however, contain medically accepted aphrodisiacal drugs in the true sense of the word. I have put an asterisk (*) after those that were considered especially powerful. In case you're interested in experimenting with any of them, I would strongly advise caution with those marked with a dagger (†), as they contain either strong drugs or corrosive and otherwise potentially poisonous properties.

Almonds
Anemones †
Anise seed
Basil
Bay leaves and seeds
Beans
Birthwort (Aristolochia Cymbifera) †
Calamint
Calamus root
Capers
Caraway seed
Cardamom
Celandine †
Celery
China root (Smilax china) †
Cloves
Coriander
Cubeb leaves and berries * (These were used extensively in Chinese and Arabian love potions.)
Cucumber
Cumin seeds
Darnel grass
Fenugreek seeds
Figs
Garlic

Ginger
Ginseng root *
Gotu kola (Hydrocotyle asiatica minor) †
Hemp *†
Hygrophilia spinosa
Ivy-leafed cyclamen root *
Jasmine flowers
Joe-pye weed (Eupatorium purpureum) †
Juniper berries
Lady's mantle (Alchemilla vulgaris) †
Lady's tresses (Spiranthes autumnales) *
Lobelia †
Lupin †
Lycopodium moss (club moss)
Maidenhair fern
Male fern (Dryopteris Felix-mas) †
Mallow
Mandrake (Atropa mandragora) †
Matico (Piper angustifolium; used in Peru as an aphrodisiac)
Mugwort
Muira puama bark †
Myrtle

Nasturtium

Nettles

Nux vomica †

Onion

Orchis satyrion root * ("Satyr's orchid" is surely an appropriate name for this herb. Salep, a Turkish aphrodisiac tea greatly in vogue during the eighteenth and nineteenth centuries in Europe, was made from its curiously shaped roots. Long after Dioscorides' day, witches continued to use them—fresh for love potions, withered for anaphrodisiac brews.)

Pansy

Parsley

Pellitory of Spain

Periwinkle

Pine nuts

Psoralea corrylifolia (An old Chinese aphrodisiac.)

Rocket cress (This herb has also been used in love potions since the days of the Romans. They used to plant it around statues of Priapus, a phallic nature god who protected gardens. Matthias L'Obel, the seventeenth-century herbalist, gives an account of how some monks once made a cordial from it, and subsequently went on a rampage among the women in the monastery's neighborhood.)

Rosemary

Roses and rose hips

Rue

Sage

Sarsaparilla

Savory

Sea holly *(eryngo)* *

Southernwood * (Apart from its use in love potions, the ashes of this herb were for a long time considered to promote the growth of hair on young men's chins if applied in ointment form.)

Spearmint

Spreading hogsweed

Tarragon

Thyme

Tormentil * (A very popular ingredient of old love charms. One such runs: "Tormentil! Tormentil! Make so-and-so subject to my will!" These words were to be chanted over the herb before it was secretly introduced into the victim's food.)

Valerian

Vervain * (An herb once sacred to the Druids. Vervain is another old favorite in love charms.)

Violet

White poppy (opium poppy, *Papaver somniferum*) †

Wild columbine (*Aquilegia*) †

254 / MASTERING HERBALISM

TRADITIONAL LOVE POTIONS

In North Africa and Asia Minor, where many of the herbalist's love secrets seem to have originated, honey is frequently added to love potions. It often appears in combination with hot resins or spices, for these were thought to stir the fires of human passion very effectively. Scammony resin and honey was one such "sure-fire" potion; gum mastic and honey another. A prototypical marzipan made of rose water, almonds, and honey was a third. A mixture of elecampane, vervain, and mistletoe berries, while not tasting so good as the others, was also a time-honored combination which often found its way into the food or drink of the unsuspecting loved one. A delicious supposedly aphrodisiac hippocras used to be brewed by steeping cinnamon, ginger, and vanilla pods in wine mixed with a little rhubarb juice. Or a fragrant powder made from ground nuts, cloves, ginger, lavender blossoms, and nutmeg could be slipped into the victim's food. A traditional aphrodisiac soup worthy of the *Arabian Nights* made from doves or any other fowl (which would presumably include chickens, for those interested in trying it) was flavored with galangal root, cardamom seeds, bay seeds, nutmeg, cubebs, and a pinch of sparrow-wort (*Erica passerina*, a type of heather). Aphrodisiac ointments to smear on the genitals and erogenous zones were also much in demand. Frankincense, myrrh, and camphor macerated in musk and rose water was one formula. Another called for ginger root, pellitory of Spain, and lilac oil. Both ginger and pellitory act as local external stimulants and rubifacients which undoubtedly accounts for their presence here. Those all-time favorites, musk, civet, and ambergris, were used in potion and perfume alike, and turned up in every possible combination. Musk has long been valued for its aphrodisiac effect, but chiefly in Iran and China; civet became the favorite perfume of any eighteenth-century rakes who took their progress seriously, and ambergris was the seductive perfume relied on by one of Louis XV's less venal mistresses, Madame du Barry.

Of course, these are only the more palatable potion ingredients. As often as not, bizarre or grotesque substances would also enter into the formulas. When obtainable, crocodile kidneys and other exotic offal, ground spiders, and the sexual organs and excreta of a variety of animals were pressed into service, their use deriving ultimately from long-discarded rites of the forgotten fertility cults.

THE REAL APHRODISIACS

But what of the real turn-ons? Considering the vast array of traditional ones, they are surprisingly few in number.

Black American Willow Bark (Salyx nigra)

OTHER NAMES. Pussy willow. Catkins willow.

HABITAT. Originally a native of the United States, pussy willow is now grown all over the world as an ornamental tree. Its black bark, lance-shaped leaves, and pretty catkins make it an obvious choice for any damp low-lying ground in gardens, especially beside ponds or rivers.

PROPERTIES. Pussy willow bark contains tannin and salinigrin, a white crystalline glucoside soluble in both water and alcohol with tonic, sedative, and aphrodisiac properties.

HOW TO USE IT. Mrs. Grieve recommends that ½ to 1 drachm of the fluid extract be taken (approximately ½ to 1 teaspoon).

Burra Gookeroo Seeds (Pedalium murex or Tribulus terrestes)

OTHER NAME. Burra gokhru.

HABITAT. This is a thorny plant indigenous to India.

PROPERTIES. Burra gookeroo seeds are considered by herbalists to possess demulcent, diuretic, and aphrodisiac properties. It is used for treating male impotence.

HOW TO USE IT. Infuse 1 part seeds in 20 parts water, and take 3 times daily. Fluid extract, 10 to 30 drops.

Cactus Flowers (Cereus grandiflorus)

OTHER NAMES. Night-blooming cereus. Vanilla cactus. Large-flowered cactus. Sweet-scented cactus.

HABITAT. United States, Mexico, the West Indies, and Naples.

256 / MASTERING HERBALISM

A fleshy shrub with cylindrical stems, clusters of typical cactus spines, and large 8- to 12-inch whitish flowers which exude a heavy vanillalike perfume at night. The flowers last only one night, and give place to gooseberrylike fruit containing an acid juice.

PROPERTIES. The cereus flowers and stems contain resins and a powerful cardiac stimulant partially similar in action to digitalis, the derivative of young foxglove leaves. In large doses it has been known to produce gastric irritation and hallucinations. Though not acting directly upon the sexual organs, cactus flowers are advocated by some herbalists in tincture or decoction form as a tonic to alleviate sexual exhaustion.

How TO USE IT. Grieve advocates 1 to 10 mimims (drops) of the liquid extract (decoction), or 2 to 30 mimims of the tincture. I need hardly add, of course, that great caution should be exercised with this herb, as with any powerful alkaloid.

Damiana Leaves (Turnera aphrodisiaca)

OTHER NAME. Mexican damiana.

HABITAT. Mexico, West Indies, California, Texas, South America. A small shrubby herb with smooth pale leaves ¼ to 1 inch long, possessing an aromatic odor when dry, and a minty taste.

PROPERTIES. Damiana contains a volatile essential oil that smells a bit like camomile; resins, tannin, and damianin, an amorphous bitter principle. Its action is mildly purgative, diuretic, stimulant, tonic, and strongly aphrodisiac, acting directly on the genital organs.

How TO USE IT. Damiana may be used in the form of a decoction or an infusion. It is sometimes prescribed by herbalists in combination with nux vomica or saw palmetto berries (q.v.).

Damiana Tea

Infuse 1 teaspoon dried damiana leaves in 1 covered cup boiling water for 15 minutes. Flavor with honey if required and drink up to 2 cups per day.

Tincture and fluid extract (decoction): ½ to 1 drachm (teaspoon).

Echinacea Root (*Echinacea angustifolia* or *Brauneria pallida*)

OTHER NAMES. Coneflower. Black sampson. Sampson root. Purple coneflower. Rudbeckia.

HABITAT. Western United States, Britain. The root of this deep-purple flower contains, among other things, resin, an oil, inulin, inuloid, sucrose, betaine, and two phytosterols.

PROPERTIES. Herbalists claim echinacea increases the body's resistance to infection. It has been used to treat boils, erysipelas, syphilis, and even cancer, although its virtues in this area are as yet unproven. It is also thought to be a powerful aphrodisiac.

HOW TO USE IT. Steep 1 teaspoon of the dried, granulated root in 1 covered cup boiling water for 30 minutes. Take 1 tablespoon strained liquid flavored with honey if required up to 6 times a day. Tincture dosage: 5 to 10 mimims (drops).

Guarana Seeds (*Paullinia cupana* or *P. sorbilis*)

OTHER NAMES. Guarana bread. Brazilian cocoa. Uaranzeiro. Uabano.

HABITAT. Uruguay and Brazil. The seeds of this climbing shrub are roasted and pounded into a fine powder. This is then mixed with water and rolled into small sticks to be dried in the sun or over a slow fire.

PROPERTIES. A bitter chocolaty drink made from grated guarana sticks, about three times as stimulating as a cup of coffee. The plant contains guaranine (identical to caffeine), tannic acid, and a green, nonvolatile oil. Herbalists use guarana as a stimulant, nervine, tonic, febrifuge, and aphrodisiac.

HOW TO USE IT. Guarana tastes best when masked by some sweeter substance such as hot chocolate or strawberry jam. Mrs. Grieve advocates using up to ½ drachm (½ teaspoon) as a simple dose. Many herbalists just stir it into the chocolate or mix it with the jam and spread it on a cookie.

Kava Kava Root (*Piper methysticum*)

OTHER NAMES. Intoxicating pepper. Ava pepper.
HABITAT. Polynesia, Pacific islands, Sandwich Islands. Kava kava

was originally eaten by the Pacific islanders as a ritual sacrament before important religious ceremonies. Although the Samoans still make use of a kava ritual, the drink has largely passed into everyday usage.

PROPERTIES. Kava kava contains an aromatic, bitter, soapy-tasting resin with the capacity of inducing sleep and a state of tranquility in the user. Taken in excess it can, like all alkaloids, prove dangerous or even fatal, for it will cause ulceration and ultimately paralyze the respiratory center. Taken in moderation however, some herbalists claim it has an aphrodisiacal effect.

HOW TO USE IT. Mrs. Grieve recommends that 1 drachm of the powdered root be taken (approximately 1 teaspoon). The easiest way to do this is in capsule form—empty caps can be obtained from some pharmacies.

Saw Palmetto (Sarenoa serrulata)

OTHER NAMES. *Sabal serrulata.* Fan palm. Dwarf palmetto.

HABITAT. Saw palmetto is a native of the southeastern seaboard of the United States. It grows to between 6 to 10 feet in height, and the red-brown, inch-long berry contains its active principle.

PROPERTIES. Diuretic, tonic, sedative, and anticatarrhal. The berries are also claimed to have a directly stimulant effect upon the breasts and the testicles.

HOW TO USE IT. Infuse 1 teaspoon dried berries in 1 covered cup boiling water for 10 minutes. Strain and flavor with honey if required. Up to 2 cold cups per day may be drunk.

Yohimbe Bark (Corynanthe yohimbine)

HABITAT. West Africa.

PROPERTIES. Yohimbe bark contains the powerful alkaloids yohimbine and yohimbiline, which in minimal doses act generally as tranquilizers, lowering blood pressure and reducing tension. In large doses, however, yohimbe causes intoxication and hallucinations. Yohimbe is probably the most well known and widely accepted organic aphrodisiac. It acts directly upon the genital organs, stimulating the spinal nerves and increasing the flow of blood to the pelvic area.

HOW TO USE IT. Opinions vary among herbalists as to the best way of making use of the aphrodisiac powers of yohimbe. One method [4] calls for simmering 5 to 8 teaspoons shaved bark or 3 to 6 teaspoons powdered bark for 5 minutes in 1 pint boiling water. The liquid should then be filtered and 1000 milligrams ascorbic acid (vitamin C, obtainable at any pharmacy) added to each cup of liquid. The ascorbic acid apparently reacts with the alkaloids to produce the salts, yohimbine and yohimbiline ascorbate, which are far more readily assimilated by the digestive tract than the plain alkaloids, which would normally have to react with the hydrochloric acid in one's own digestive juices.

Another method [5] calls for encapsulating 1 ounce of powdered Yohimbe bark into 00 gelatin capsules and taking three at a time when required.

Although users of Yohimbe claim the drug is not addicting and has no harmful side-effects, it is a powerful one, and should be treated cautiously. It should never, on any account, be taken in conjunction with alcohol, as this combination is said to be extremely toxic.

[4] See *Herbal Aphrodisiacs*, by M. J. Superweed (San Francisco: Stone Kingdom Syndicate, 1970).

[5] See *Herbs and Things*, by Jeanne Rose (New York: Grosset and Dunlap, 1972).

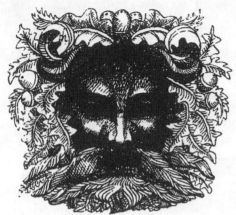

6

WITCHCRAFT
AND
WORTCUNNING

IMAGINE YOURSELF STANDING IN SOME dark forest in Europe ten centuries ago. All around you the wide trunks of trees stretch up into the golden-green ceiling of leaves overhead; beneath your feet lies a thick carpet of dead leaves—hundreds of centuries of leaves. Examine the trees on either side of you. There grows the smooth pale trunk of a holly bush, tall and many-branched and stately; its dark, prickly leaves contrasting vividly with the delicate pale-green keys of the ash tree which grows beyond it. And there, on the other side of you grows a vast, spreading oak, its trunk gray and wrinkled, gnarled by many centuries; its widely spreading branches each as thick as a lesser tree, heavy with clusters of acorns.

This was once a Druid wood, but though the Druids and the Romans have now been gone for many centuries, the trees remain, the oak, the ash and the thorn, the guardians of Britain, tall, silent, impressive, ancient, and very powerful. Why should people like the Rhizotomists and the Druids have revered these inanimate objects? Was it solely on account of their curative properties? What is this power that even today we feel lurking in trees? Merely atavistic superstitious awe?

Up until very recently any self-respecting scientist or anyone else possessed of plain common sense would have unequivocally answered "yes." People invest awesome inanimate objects—stones, trees, and the heavenly bodies—with personalities and worship them in an effort to coerce them to provide good crops, rain,

260

fertility, or whatever else they require. Such beliefs are called animism. If the tree possessed curative properties—the oak leaves are rich in tannin, and those of the holly and ash are febrifuges—then they were so much the more powerful as gods. I say up until recently, because the case seems to be a little different today.

Remarkable experiments recently conducted first by Cleve Backster and later repeated by other investigators, both in the United States and in the Soviet Union, have indicated that plants may well possess "emotions" of their own, even personalities. In 1966, Backster, a former polygraph expert with the C.I.A. who runs his own School of Lie Detection in New York, conceived the idea of hooking a plant up to one of his lie detectors, machines which measure a body's change in conductivity. Backster discovered to his surprise that the plant registered no response to any *physical* action he performed upon it, but did register one to the apparent *thought* of violence, in this instance the threat of burning. Recent Soviet investigations have topped Backster's extraordinary discoveries. Plants have been found to respond at a distance to violent emotions suggested to a hypnotized subject!

Backster's experiments and those of the Russians suggest that plants possess not only rudimentary personalities of some sort, but personalities that are capable of responding to the emotions of human beings in their vicinity. Of course, seasoned gardeners have known this for years. A friend of mine recently impaled his hand on a large thorn while planting a rosebush and, experiencing a sudden burst of hatred for the offending bush, cursed it violently. The rose wilted steadily over the next few days, while the other bushes planted at the same time did well. Only after being presented with an abject apology and some genuinely heartfelt kind words of encouragement at my instigation did the rose finally begin to pull itself together. I'm quite sure it would have died if my friend hadn't performed what seemed to him at the time an extremely foolish and superstitious action. Most gardeners have tales like this to tell. We don't even have to recount the biblical story of Jesus cursing the fig tree to demonstrate the power of human thought over plants. We all know people who have "green thumbs." They apparently have a built-in sympathy for plants, and at their touch plants seem to bloom more prolifically.

Ancient herbalists undoubtedly understood this phenomenon

very well, for they always related to their plants on a personal level. Most of their plant lore was tied up in a framework of religious or magical beliefs, some fragments of which we still come across in the older herbals. In the introduction I mentioned the practices of the Rhizotomists. This occult fraternity continued to practice its old herbal magic well into the fourth century after Christ. From what we know of their beliefs, they were practically identical with those of both the Druids and the old Roman herbalists mentioned by Pliny. It is these Romano-Celtic beliefs, combined with those of the Saxon and Teutonic tribes, that survived among European village witches from the eleventh century on. Witches, or "cunning-folk," as they came to be known in England, preserved many of the ancient pagan customs, such as the midsummer and midwinter fires, the sword dances and May rites, usually forgetting the religious reasons that had once lain behind them. Sir James Frazer recounts one Scottish incident of how the secret of lighting a midsummer fire was vested in the village wizard. The cunning-folk also practiced clairvoyance—they divined the identity of thieves in magic mirrors; and conjured up spirits to look for buried treasures. Undoubtedly they would be called psychics today. Cattle curing was also performed, and of course healing with herbs, or "wortcunning," was a major concern.

As any witch can tell you (for they still exist), herbs sometimes do their work best if you talk to them first, persuade them to act on your behalf. Don't laugh. This is only an extension of the "green thumb" principle. Herbs seem to act as resonators or thought batteries. They absorb, react to, and reflect emotions and ideas, as Mr. Backster has recently demonstrated. This surely explains why a pagan or medieval witch would always "enchant" an herb before picking and administering it. That is, she would address it, state what she wanted it for, and ask its assistance, quite matter-of-factly. She would then (I say she—it could just as well be he) usually fill the hole left by the herb, if she had dug it up, with a little gift to Mother Earth, usually wine, milk, a little corn or bread, or honey, often in the form of hydromel. Naturally, the nonbeliever is perfectly entitled to his opinion that this was all superstitious mumbo-jumbo designed to influence the credulous, and to suggest to the patient that he get well. There is a lot to be said for this. Suggestion plays a large part. But in my opinion there is and was much more to the practice than simple suggestion. The phenomenon of extrasensory perception is difficult for the unbiased observer to dismiss, and if a psychically gifted person can pick up impressions surrounding a material object (such as the knife used in a murder), then, conversely, objects can surely be consciously impressed with emotions and ideas too. And if the object—an herb—possesses some degree of life of its own which has *also* been aligned with the intention to cure, then how much better its chances of doing so. An herb enchanted in this manner—"enchanted" means simply "sung to"—was known as an amulet.

Most of the old rural witches' spell books still in circulation, such as the *Long Lost Friend* and the *Secrets of Albertus Magnus*, give many prescriptions for amulets of various kinds, herbal and otherwise. If any of these old amulets were to be anything more than ridiculous relics, they would require some sort of emotional "charging" beforehand. The process for doing this was an elaborate one. You had to work up the appropriate emotional head of steam, as it were. Where and when the rules originated is anybody's guess. However, the traditional prohibition against the use of iron or steel does point to an extremely ancient derivation, possibly in the Bronze Age and maybe even the Stone Age.

Traditional Herb-gathering Rules

From what we can gather from Pliny and other ancient herbal texts, there was a definite ritual to be adopted when gathering and "charging" herbs, which, though differing in minor details, seems to have been consistent throughout Europe.

1. Pluck herbs with the left hand. When the right hand is used, it must be poked furtively out through the loose left sleeve of the robe, pickpocket fashion, for the less Mother Earth knows about what is going on the better!

2. Never face into the wind when plucking an herb.

3. Never glance behind you.

4. Never touch the herb with cold iron. If a circle is to be drawn around the herb with a sword or knife, as is sometimes required, the blade should not be allowed to touch the roots. Anything but iron should be used to cut the plant, as iron destroys all ancient magic.

Deer horn, bronze (in the form of a knife, a sickle, or even a sharpened coin), wood, stone, even gold (the Druids used this) can be employed, but never iron or steel.

5. Always address the herb as you cut it and tell it what you are going to do with it. There are a variety of old rhymes which can be used for this purpose.

6. Never let the herb touch the ground once it has been picked, or its power will leak back into the earth again. Use a cloth or basket to lay it in. Pliny tells us that many old herbalists used to retain a portion of the herbs they sold. If they didn't receive payment, they would replant this portion, thus "discharging" the sold part.

7. Ideally, although witches tend less and less to follow this most important rule, you must wear either white linen and no shoes or no clothes at all when you pluck the herb. No jewelry should be worn either. Also, more power can be infused into the herb if the operator fasts and refrains from sexual contact for a day or two beforehand. No doubt these observances help to reinforce the concentration which is necessary to "impress" the plant and turn it into a psychic battery.

8. Finally, the earth has to be rewarded with a little gift of some sort, usually an offering of wine, honey, mead, hydromel, bread, corn, or a small coin.

Astrological conditions sometimes have to be observed, such as the state of the moon or the relative position of the planets. Most of the old writers agree that amulet herbs—herbs used as psychic batteries—are best plucked sometime at night, usually around sunset, midnight, or sunrise.

The Druids observed most of these rules. They seem to have revered plant life in general, but particularly the mistletoe and the tree it is most commonly found growing upon in Europe, the oak. The oak and the ash and the holly, the three trees commonly planted in the sacred groves of the Druids, have continued to be revered down through the centuries. In Celtic countries they remained trees on which oaths were sworn such as that taken by the legendary Scottish hero Glasgerion: "Glasgerion swore a full great oath, By Oak and Ash, and Thorn." Rudyard Kipling wove them into his romance of ancient magic, *Puck of Pook's Hill* on this account. That the Druids practiced a form of vegetation cult, as Pliny suggests, is corroborated by the traditions of the medieval Welsh bards, who by their own testimony were the inheritors of quite a bit of Druidic lore. The "Cad Goddeu," or "Battle of the Trees," a mysterious thirteenth-century poem attributed to a bard called Taliesin, recounts how the ancient Celtic gods of light overcame those of darkness with the assistance of the trees and herbs which Gwydion, the Celtic Woden, summoned by his magic. Included in the helpful array conjured up were the alder, the willow, the rowan, the plum; the medlar, the bean, the raspberry, the privet; the woodbine, the ivy, the gorse, the cherry; the birch, the pine, the elm, the hazel; the mulberry, the beech, the holly, the poplar; the fern, the furze, the heather, the black cherry; the gloomy ash—and, of course, the oak "swiftly moving" before whom heaven and earth tremble!

Saxon Wortcunning

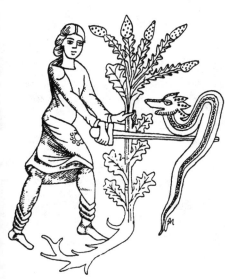

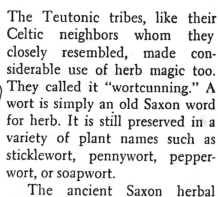

The Teutonic tribes, like their Celtic neighbors whom they closely resembled, made considerable use of herb magic too. They called it "wortcunning." A wort is simply an old Saxon word for herb. It is still preserved in a variety of plant names such as sticklewort, pennywort, pepperwort, or soapwort.

The ancient Saxon herbal known as *The Lacnunga* contains the following herb incantation. It refers to nine different plants, each considered useful for healing a different type of malady. You will recognize most of them from Chapter 1. Whenever the Saxon herbalist wished to administer one, he would chant the relevant portion of the verse over it.

WORMWOOD, A
SERPENT-ROUTING HERB
(after an Anglo-Saxon herbal)

THE NINE-HERBS CHARM

Forget not, Mugwort, what thou didst reveal,
What thou didst prepare at Regenmeld.
Thou hast strength against three and against thirty,
Thou hast strength against poison and against infection,
Thou hast strength against the foe who fares through the land!

And thou, Plantain, Mother of herbs,
Open from the East, mighty within,
Over thee chariots creaked, over thee queens rode,
Over thee brides made outcry, over thee bulls gnashed their teeth.
All these thou didst withstand and resist;
So mayest thou withstand poison and infection,
And the foe who fares through the land!

This herb is called Stime;[1] it grew on a stone,
It resists poison, it fights pain.
It is called harsh, it fights against poison.
This is the herb that strove with the snake;
This has strength against poison, this has strength against infection,
This has strength against the foe who fares through the land!

Now, Cock's-spur Grass,[2] conquer the greater poisons, though thou
    art the lesser;
Thou, the mightier, vanquish the lesser until he is cured of both!

Remember, Mayweed,[3] what thou didst reveal
What thou didst bring to pass at Alford:
That he never yielded his life because of infection,
After Mayweed was dressed for his food!

[1] Watercress, particularly valuable for its antiscorbutic properties and mineral content. At one time it was considered a specific for tuberculosis.

[2] *Cynadon dactylon*. Still used by French herbalists as a diaphoretic and demulcent.

[3] Camomile.

This is the herb which is called Wergulu;[4]
The seal sent this over the back of the ocean
To heal the hurt of other poison!

These nine sprouts against nine poisons.
A snake came crawling, it bit a man
Then Woden took nine glory-twigs,
Smote the serpent so that it flew into nine parts,
There Apple [5] brought this to pass against poison,
That she nevermore would enter her house!

Thyme [6] and Fennel, a pair great in power,
The Wise Lord,[7] holy in heaven,
Wrought these herbs while He hung on the cross;
He placed and put them in the seven worlds to aid all, poor and rich.

It stands against pain, resists the venom,
It has power against three and against thirty,
Against a fiend's hand and against sudden trick,
Against witchcraft of vile creatures!

Now these nine herbs avail against nine evil spirits,
Against nine poisons and against nine infectious diseases,
Against the red poison, against the running poison,
Against the yellow poison, against the green poison,
Against the black poison, against the dark poison,
Against snake-blister, against water-blister,
Against thorn-blister, against thistle-blister,
Against ice-blister, against poison-blister,
If any poison comes flying from the east or any comes from the north,
Or any from the west upon the people.

[4] Nettle, "Urtica urens" or "dioica."

[5] An apple a day keeps the doctor away, I suppose.

[6] Some scholars translate this as Chervil, rather than Thyme.

[7] "The Wise Lord" could refer to either Christ or Woden here. Woden hung himself on the World Tree to gain magic knowledge of runes, slips of wood used for divination by the Saxons and Teutons.

Christ stood over disease of every kind.
I alone know running water,[8] and the nine serpents heed it;
May all pastures now spring up with herbs,
The seas, all salt water, be destroyed,
When I blow this poison from thee!

Another ancient charm used by the Saxons runs as follows. It was used to ask Mother Earth to give them good herbs and crops:

> Erce, Erce, Erce, Mother of Earth!
> May the All-Wielder, Ever Lord grant thee
> Acres a-waxing, upwards a-growing
> Pregnant [with corn] and plenteous in strength;
> Hosts of [grain] shafts and of glittering plants!
> And of white wheat ears waxing,
> Of the whole earth the harvest!
> Let be guarded the grain against all ills
> That are sown o'er the land by the sorcery men [9]
> Nor let the cunningwoman change it nor crafty man.[10]

Medieval Herb Magic

By the advent of the eleventh and twelfth centuries in Europe, most of the old pagan religious practices were all but replaced by Christian variants. Old festivals had been whitewashed and turned into saints' days. The "cunning-folk" of rural communities now called on Jesus, Mary, and the saints in their herbal charms. Occasionally, however, heathen elements did remain, unrecognized and therefore unmolested, as in the following impressive spell used by twelfth-century herbalists. Here the earth is invoked as a mother in time-honored fashion. She is even addressed as "goddess," which is extraordinary, considering the growing climate of suspicion and persecution of heresy:

[8] A very ancient antiwitch specific.
[9] In today's terms, the ecological bandits no doubt.
[10] The evil witch and wizard.

Earth,[11] divine goddess, Mother Nature who generatest all things and bringest forth anew the sun which thou hast given to the nations; Guardian of sky and sea and of all gods and powers . . . through thy power all nature falls silent and then sinks in sleep. And again thou bringest back the light and chasest away night and yet again thou coverest us most securely with thy shades. Thou dost contain chaos infinite, yea and winds and showers and storms; thou sendest them out when thou wilt and causest the seas to roar; thou chasest away the sun and arousest the storm. Again when thou wilt thou sendest forth the joyous day and givest the nourishment of life with thy eternal surety; and when the soul departs to thee we return. Thou indeed art duly called great Mother of the Gods; thou conquerest by thy divine name. Thou art the source of the strength of nations and of gods, without thee nothing can be brought to perfection or be born; thou art great queen of the gods. Goddess! I adore thee as divine; I call upon thy name; be pleased to grant that which I ask thee, so shall I give thanks to thee, Goddess, with due faith.

Hear, I beseech thee, and be favorable to my prayer. Whatsoever herb thy power dost produce, give, I pray, with goodwill to all nations to save them and grant me this my medicine. Come to me with thy powers, and howsoever I may use them may they have good success and to whomsoever I may give them. Whatever thou dost grant it may prosper. To thee all things return. Those who rightly receive these herbs from me, do thou make them whole. Goddess, I beseech thee; I pray thee as a suppliant that by thy majesty thou grant this to me.

Now I make intercession to you all ye powers and herbs and to your majesty, ye whom Earth parent of all hath produced and given as a medicine of health to all nations and hath put majesty upon you, I pray you, the greatest help to the human race. This I pray and beseech from you, and be present here with your virtues, for she who created you hath herself promised that I may gather you into the goodwill of him on whom the art of medicine was bestowed, and grant for health's sake good medicine by grace of your powers. I pray grant me through your virtues that whatsoe'er is wrought by me

---

[11] Translation from "Early English Magic and Medicine" by Dr. Charles Singer, *Proceedings of the British Academy,* Vol. IV.

through you may in all its powers have a good and speedy effect and
good success and that I may always be permitted with the favor of
your majesty to gather you into my hands and to glean your fruits.
So shall I give thanks to you in the name of that majesty which
ordained your birth!

Albertus Magnus, a prolific thirteenth-century scholar and
student of the occult, included a paragraph on magical herb
gathering in one of his many books. He advocated plucking herbs
governed by the seven planets during the last quarter of the moon.
Instead of laying the plucked herb upon the druidic white cloth, he
recommends using wheat or barley.

Yet this is to be marked, that these hearbs [12] be gathered from
the three and twentieth day of the Moone, until the thirti[e]th day
beginning the Signe Mercurius by the space of a whole house. And in
gathering make mention of the passion or greefe, and the name of
the thing for the which thou dost gather it, and the selfe hearb.
Notwithstanding, lay the hearb upon wheat or barley, and use it
afterwards unto thy uses.

Three hundred years later, many of the old practices were still in
use. Thomas Tusser, writing in 1573, advises:
Sowe peason and beanes, in the wane of the moone,
Who soweth them sooner, he soweth too soone,
That they with the planet may rest and arise,
And flourish, with bearing most plentiful wise!
This, of course, is nothing but ancient moon lore purged of its
paganism. Old ways are hard to change. Names are easy. Charms
were still spoken over herbs, but they were now more in the nature
of prayers. All overt references to pagan gods had now been
replaced by Christian invocations.

Now Calvary, the hill upon which Christ was crucified and the
site of old Eden, was often named as the place where the wonder-
working herb first grew, as in this sixteenth-century herb-culling
charm:

---

[12] Assodilius, poligonia, chynostates' plantain, cinquefoil, henbane, vervain.

Haile be thou, holie herbe, growing on the ground
All in the mount Calvarie first wert thou found.
Thou art good for manie a sore, and healest many a wound;
In the name of sweet Jesus, I take thee from the ground!

An even simpler French charm conjured the wild herb with these words:

Sacred herb, which hast neither been sowed, nor planted, show forth the power God has given thee!

Seventeenth-century Herb Magic

The last of the occult herbalists, Nicholas Culpeper, included the following instructions to the would-be astrological herb gatherer who intended to harvest his herbs when the planets that ruled them formed harmonious aspects with one another.

Let the planet that governs the herb be angular, and the stronger the better; [that is, let it be in the first, fourth, seventh, or tenth house of the horoscope] if they can, in herbs of Saturn, let Saturn be in the ascendant; in the herb of Mars, let Mars be in the Mid-heaven, for in those houses they delight; let the Moon apply to them by good aspect [that is, in conjunction, trine, or sextile] and let her not be in the houses of her enemies [i.e., in modern astrological terms, she should not be in her fall or detriment]; if you cannot well stay till she apply to them [get into a good aspect] let her apply to a planet of the same triplicity; if you cannot wait that time neither, let her be with a fixed star of their nature.

Having well dried them, put them up in brown paper, sewing the paper up like a sack, and press them not too hard together, and keep them in a dry place near the fire . . .

Culpeper's Astrological Herbs

HERBS RULED BY SATURN

(That is, herbs considered by Culpeper to be anodyne, bitter, funereal, melancholic, or otherwise Saturnine.)

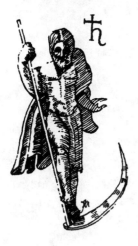

Aconite
Amaranth
Barley
Beech tree
Beet
Birdsfoot
Bucks horn plantain
Buckthorn
Campion
Comfrey
Cress
Crosswort
Cypress

Darnel
Dodder
Elm
Osmond royal fern
Flea wort
Fluxweed
Fumitory
Oak gall
Gladiolus
Gladwin
Goat herb
Hawkweed
Heartsease
Hellebore
Hemlock
Hemp
Henbane
Holly
Horsetail
Ivy
Jew's ear
Juniper
Knapweed
Knapwort
Knot grass

Meadow saffron
Medlar
Mullein
Navelwort
Nightshade
Poplar
Quince
Ragwort
Root of scarcity
Rupturewort
Rush
Safflower
Sciatica grass
Service tree
Shepherd's purse
Sloe
Solomon's seal
Tamarisk
Thorough leaf
Thrift
Tutsan
Water violet
Willow herb
Woad
Yew

HERBS RULED BY JUPITER

(Herbs considered soothing, cheering, benevolent, and otherwise Jovial.)

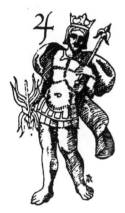

Avens
Balm
Betony
Bilberry
Borage
Box
Briar rose
Chervil
Chestnut
Cinquefoil
Costmary
Currant
Agrimony   Dandelion
Alexander   Dock
Asparagus   Couch grass

Eglantine
Endive
Fig tree
Fir tree
Goat's beard
Gold of pleasure
Golden samphire
Hart's tongue
House leek
Hyssop
Jasmine
Oxtongue
Sea lightwort
Lime tree
Liverwort

Lungwort
Maple tree
Meadowsweet
Myrrh
Whitlow grass
Oak
Pinks
Polypody fern
Sage
Scurvy grass
Succory
Sumac
Swallow wort
Thorn apple
Thorough wax

HERBS RULED BY MARS

(Herbs considered sharp, acrid, biting, sour, or irritant.)

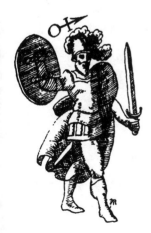

Anemone
Arssmart
Asarabaca
Barberry
Basil
Black cress
Briony
Broom
Butcher's broom
Cotton thistle

Crowfoot
Cuckoo pint
Eveweed
Felwort
Flaxweed
Furze
Galangal
Garlic
Gentian
Germander

Hawthorn
Holy thistle
Honeysuckle
Hops
Horse tongue
Hedge hyssop
Lupin
Madder
Masterwort
Mastic herb
Mustard
Nettle
Onion

Parsley
Pepper
Pine
Radish
Rest harrow
Rhubarb
Rocket
Saltwort
Samphire
Sanicle
Sarsaparilla
Savine
Shepherd's rod

Simson
Sowbread
Sowerweed
Spurge
Squill
Tarragon
Tobacco
Toothcress
Woodruff
Wormseed
Wormwood

HERBS RULED BY THE SUN

(Herbs considered fragrant, royal, holy, or sun-seeking.)

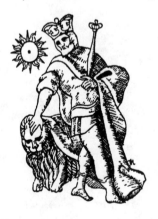

Angelica
Ash tree
Bay
Burnet
Butter-bur
Camomile
Celandine
Centaury
Eyebright
Heart trefoil
Heliotrope
Honey-wort
Lovage
Marigold

Mistletoe
Peony
Rice
Rosemary
Rue
Saffron
St. John's wort
Storax
Sundew
Tormentil
Vine
Viper's bugloss
Wake Robin
Walnut

HERBS RULED BY VENUS

(Herbs considered sweet, fragrant, delicious, aphrodisiac, or cosmetic.)

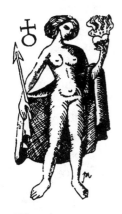

Alkanet
Alder, black
Alder, common
Bean
Birch
Bishop's weed
Blackberry
Blites
Bugle
Burdock
Catnip
Cherry
Chickpease
Cock's head
Coltsfoot
Columbine
Cowslip
Crab's claws

Cudweed
Daffodil
Daisy
Dittany of Crete
Elder
Eryngo
Feverfew
Figwort
Foxglove
Fraxinella
Geranium
Goldenrod
Gooseberry
Gosmore
Groundsel
Kidneywort
Ladies bedstraw
Ladies mantel
Lentils
Mallow
Mint
Moneywort
Motherwort
Mugwort
Orach
Orchis
Peach
Pear

Pennyroyal
Pennywort
Pepperwort
Periwinkle
Plantain
Plowman's spikenard
Plum
Poley
Primrose
Rampion
Raspberry
Rose
Self-heal
Shepherd's needle
Sicklewort
Skirret
Soapwort
Sow thistle
Speedwell
Spignel
Strawberry
Sycamore
Tansy
Thyme
Vervain
Violet
Woodsage
Yarrow

HERBS RULED BY MERCURY

(Herbs thought to induce internal activity. Mercury rules "movement.")

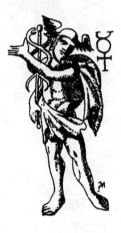

Calamint
Caraway
Dill
Elecampane
Fennel
Fenugreek
Flax
Good King Henry
Hare's foot
Hazel
Honey-wort
Horehound
Hound's tongue
Lavender
Lavender cotton
Lily of the valley
Licorice
Maidenhair

Mandrake
Marjoram
Mulberry
Mushroom
Myrtle
Pellitory
Pomegranate
Quick grass
Savory
Scabious
Senna
Smallage
Southernwood
Spurge
Starwort
Trefoil
Valerian

HERBS RULED BY THE MOON

(Herbs considered to be cooling, drying, sleep-inducing, or otherwise "lunar.")

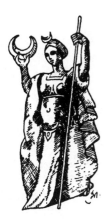

Acanthus
Adders tongue
Arrach
Chickweed
Clary

Cleavers
Coleworts, sea
Cucumber
Dog's tooth violet
Duckweed
Dwarf rocket cress
Faverel
Fluellein
French mercury
Iris
Lettuce
Lily
Moonwort
Orpine

Pearl trefoil
Poppy
Privet
Purslane
Saxifrage
Stonecrop
Touchwood
Turnip
Wallflower
Watercress
Water lily
Willow
Wintergreen
Yellow flag

Culpeper's successors have steered clear of his combination of herbalism and astrology for the most part. So, too, with the advent of eighteenth-century rationalism did the magical use of herbs become less and less a matter of common practice. But the beliefs lingered on nonetheless, in the country districts of both Europe and the United States. Jakob Grimm's *Teutonic Mythology* gives us a good look at nineteenth-century magical herbal beliefs in Europe, while the *Journal of the English Folklore Society* is full of snippets of traditional British lore. Vance Randolph's *Ozark Superstitions* provides ample evidence of the continuance of American herb-magic traditions.

This chapter would surely be incomplete without a glance at some of this fascinating lore.

A Witch's Herbal

HERBS USED TO EXORCISE EVIL SPIRITS AND NEUTRALIZE HEXES

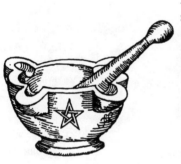

Amulet herbs were carried by the person who felt in need of protection from supernatural evil, or were hung up in some central place—over the entrance, bed, or hearth, or in the rafters. They were often tied in a bunch with red twine or wool, a practice dating back to the time of the Babylonians. The color red is the color of fire and blood, both considered very powerful things from a magical point of view.

ANGELICA. Wear or hang up as an amulet.

ASAFOETIDA GRASS. The medieval grimoire known as *The Greater Key of Solomon* advocates using this pungent herb or the resin derived from it as an incense to exorcise, that is, to call to account or banish, evilly disposed spirits.

AVENS (*Geum urbanum*). An astringent clove-tasting herb still used by herbalists as a blood-purifying infusion to aid skin complaints. However, cunning-folk have used herb bennet, as it is also called, for centuries as an amulet. The *Ortus Sanitatis*, an herbal printed in 1491 states:

"Where the root is in the house, Satan can do nothing and flies from it, wherefore it is blessed before all other herbs, and if a man carries the root about him no venomous beast can harm him."

BALDMONEY (*Gentiana amarella*). Wear or hang up as an amulet.

BAY. "Neither witch nor devil, thunder nor lightning will hurt a man in the place where a bay tree is."

BETONY. According to old herb lore, betony is "good whether for the man's soul or for his body; it shields him against visions and dreams, and the wort is very wholesome, and thus thou shalt gather it, in the month of August without the use of iron; and when thou hast gathered it, shake the mold till nought of it cleave thereon, and then dry it in the shade very thoroughly, and with its roots altogether reduce it to dust: then use it and take of it when thou needst."

BITTERSWEET, *or woody nightshade.* Hang up as an amulet.

DILL. Wear or hang this up as an amulet. One old rune says:

> Trefoil, vervain, John's wort, dill,
> Hinder witches of their will!

ELDER. Wear or hang up as an amulet. The wood should be gathered with a bare head, folded arms, and partly bended knees, while saying these words: "Lady Ellhorn, give me some of thy wood, and I will give thee some of mine when it grows in the forest!"

FENNEL. Wear or hang up as an amulet.

FRANKINCENSE AND MYRRH. Burn as an incense to exorcise spooks.

FUMITORY. Burn as an incense.

GARLIC. Wear or hang up as an amulet.

HOREHOUND, WHITE. Wear or hang up as an amulet.

HYSSOP. Wear or hang up as an amulet.

LAVENDER. Burn as an incense on Midsummer Eve.

MISTLETOE. Wear or hang up as an amulet. Mistletoe should be cut either on Midsummer's Eve, "when the sun and moon stand in the sign of their might," or on the sixth day of the moon, preferably with a gold or bronze sickle, although many present-day witches use Solomon's white-handled knife (about which more later). Like all amulet herbs, mistletoe should not be permitted to touch the ground once it is cut.

MOTHERWORT. A fifteenth-century English translation of the tenth-century Latin poem known as "Macer's Herbal" calls this herb all-powerful against "wykked sperytis."

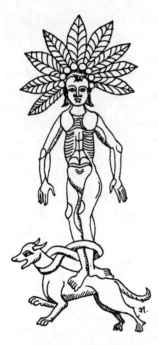

GATHERING A MANDRAKE
(after an Anglo-Saxon
herbal)

MUGWORT. Traditionally, an amulet against the evil eye, among other things.

MULLEIN. Wear or hang up as an amulet.

PEONY. A solar amulet to dispel bugaboos and nightmares. Its roots should be made into beads to hang around the neck. Classical herbalists used to tie the stem to a dog and induce it to drag the plant from the ground in a manner similar to the way they gathered mandrakes. Gerard recommended that fifteen peony seeds gathered when the moon was waning be infused in wine or mead as "a speciall remedie for those that are troubled in the night with the disease called Night Mare"!

PERIWINKLE. The 1480 edition of Apuleius' *Herbarium* has this to say about the periwinkle:

This wort is of good advantage for many purposes, that is to say, first against devil sickness and demoniacal possessions and against snakes and wild beasts and against poisons and for various wishes and for envy and for terror and that thou mayest have grace, and if thou hast the wort with thee thou shalt be prosperous and ever acceptable. This wort thou shalt pluck thus, saying:

I pray thee, vinca pervinca,
thee that art to be had for thy many useful qualities,
that thou come to me glad blossoming with thy mainfulness,
that thou outfit me so that I be shielded and ever prosperous
and undamaged by poisons and by water.

When thou shalt pluck this wort thou shalt be clean of every uncleanness, and thou shalt pick it when the moon is nine nights old and eleven nights and thirteen nights and thirty nights and when it is one night old.

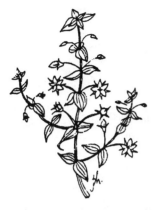

PIMPERNEL

(*Anagallis arvensis*)

PIMPERNEL *(Anagallis arvensis)*. "No heart can think, no tongue can tell the virtues of the pimpernel," says one old herbal rhyme, indicating the extraordinary reputation this little field flower once had among herbalists as a cure-all. Although modern herbalists are less enthusiastic about it nowadays, it is still used cautiously from time to time as a rheumatism and liver medicine. White witches, however, have always made good use of it. "The herb pimpernel is good to prevent witchcraft, as Mother Bumby doth affirm," says one old writer. Mother Bumby certainly knew her herb lore, for the great Solomon himself advocated the use of pimpernel to make a white-handled knife with which to cut amulet herbs. It is obviously the descendant of the bronze or gold sickle, although the once-imperative stricture against using iron on plants seems to have been relaxed. Possibly the fact that the knife was made under a good Martial aspect in the waxing moon and in the day and hour of Mercury was enough to prevent the iron from doing its usual destructive work. Unlike its black-handled twin, the white-handled knife was used to make benevolent magic rather than threatening.

King Solomon's White-handled Knife

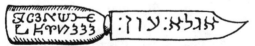

The Knife with the white hilt should be made in the day and hour of Mercury,[13] when Mars is in the Sign of the Ram or the Scorpion.[14] It should be dipped in the blood of a gosling and in the juice of the pimpernel, the Moon being at her full or increasing in light. Dip therein also the white hilt, upon which thou shalt have engraved the characters shown . . . With this Knife thou mayest perform all the necessary Operations of the Art, except the Circle . . . and thou shalt place it thrice in the fire until it becometh red-hot,

[13] See note 19.

[14] Mars traditionally exerts its strongest influence in these signs.

282 / MASTERING HERBALISM

and each time thou shalt immerse it in the aforesaid blood and juice, fasten thereunto the white hilt having engraved thereon the aforesaid characters, and upon the hilt thou shalt write with the pen of Art,[15] commencing from the point and going towards the hilt, these Names . . . when it is finished thou shalt say:

"I conjure thee, O Instrument of Steel, by God the Father Almighty, by the Virtue of the Heavens, of the Stars, and of the Angels who preside over them; by the virtue of stones, herbs, and animals; by the virtue of hail, snow, and wind; that thou receivest such virtue that thou mayest obtain without deceit the end which I desire in all things where I shall use thee; through God the Creator of the Ages, and Emperor of the Angels. Amen."

Afterwards repeat Psalms III; IX; XXXI; XLII; LX; LI; CXXX.[16] Perfume it with the perfumes of the Art,[17] and sprinkle it with exorcised water, wrap it in silk and say:

"DANI, ZUMECH, AGALMATUROD, GADIEL, PANI, CANELOAS, MEROD, GAMIDOI, BALDOI, METRATOR, Angels most holy, be present for a guard unto this instrument."

PURSLANE. This should be strewn on beds as a guard against nightmares and general ill luck.

ROWAN TREE OR MOUNTAIN ASH. A tree prized in Celtic countries from the time of the Druids onward for its protective powers against spooks, demons, and malefic witchery. The amulet should be made from two twigs tied crosswise by red wool or thread with these words:

> Black-luggie, hammer-head,[18]
> Rowan-tree, and red thread
> Put the warlocks to their speed!

ST. JOHN'S WORT. The Latin name of this herb, *Hypericum*,

[15] A sharpened goose quill blessed with the words, "ADRAI, HAHLII, TAMAII, TILONAS, ATHAMAS, ZIANOR, ADONAI, banish from this pen all deceit and error, so that it may be of virtue and efficacy to write all that I desire. Amen." The pen is then perfumed in incense smoke and sprinkled with holy water.

[16] The so-called Seven Penitential Psalms.

[17] An incense composed of lignum aloes, nutmeg, benzoin, and musk. It actually smells very good as an ordinary incense, but you must use nutmeg *oil*, not powder.

[18] Some versions of this charm read "lammer-bead," that is, amber bead. Both hammers and amber beads were considered strong preservatives from sorcery, as it happens. Black luggie is probably blackthorn.

derives from the Greek, meaning "holding power over spirits." It should be hung up on Midsummer's Eve and burned as a fumigation on the midsummer bonfire to secure its major protective properties.

SNAPDRAGON *(Antirrhinum magus)*. Wear or hang up as an amulet.

TOADFLAX *(Linaria vulgaris)*. Wear or hang up as an amulet.

VERVAIN. As magical an herb as St. John's wort, vervain had to be gathered with the left hand at the rise of the dog star, Sirius, "without being looked upon either by the sun or moon," and the earth propitiated with a gift of honey. *The Greater Key of Solomon*, however, recommends that its powers be used in the following manner:

> Thou shalt then make unto thy self a Sprinkler of vervain, fennel, lavender, sage, valerian, mint, garden-basil, rosemary, and hyssop, gathered in the day and hour of Mercury,[19] the Moon being in her increase [waxing]. Bind together these herbs with a thread spun by a young maiden, and engrave upon the handle the following characters.

topside   *underside*

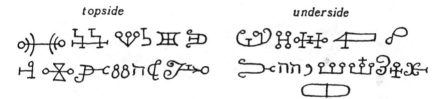

> After this thou mayest use the [holy] Water, using the Sprinkler whenever it is necessary; and know that wheresoever thou shalt sprinkle this Water, it will chase away all Phantoms, and they shall be unable to hinder or annoy thee.

LUCK-BRINGING HERBS

A wide variety of herbs were thought to actively bring luck to the bearer rather than simply to protect him from evil. They were

---

[19] Wednesday at 6 A.M., 1 P.M., or 8 P.M. according to the *Key;* 1 A.M., 8 A.M., 3 P.M., or 10 P.M. according to the other grimoires.

usually worn in rings or hung around the neck. Here are a few of the more popular ones:

CLOVER, OR TREFOIL. The four-leafed variety has always been considered especially lucky. As the old rhyme says:
>One leaf is for fame,
>And one leaf is for wealth,
>And one for a faithful lover,
>And one to bring you glorious health,
>And all in a four-leafed Clover!

FERN. Male fern root, or *Dryopteris Felix-mas*, has also been considered a potent luck-bringing amulet for many centuries, especially when its stems are cut off in such a way as to suggest fingers. Traditionally a "lucky hand" of this sort should be dried over the smoke of a midsummer bonfire first.

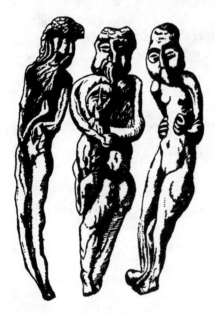

CARVED MANDRAKE AMULETS
discovered at
Antioch and Damascus

HOUSELEEK. Hang this in your rafters to keep your house from being struck by lightning.

MANDRAKE. *Mandragora officinalis* and *Bryonia dioica* both go by this name. Both of their roots were made into luck and fertility amulets during the Middle Ages. The mandrake root had to be pulled up during the waxing moon in spring. The older writers advocated using a dog to perform this action because of the belief that the shriek the mandrake root gave as it left the ground would strike the hearer dead. The root should be carved into the shape of a doll and, according to some accounts, dried over a fire made of vervain leaves.

OAK. The oak was considered by the Romans to be sacred to Jupiter, king of the gods. The Druids also held it in high esteem.

Witches, being the inheritors of much pagan lore, continued to look on it with awe and reverence. A cross of oak twigs bound with red yarn used to be enchanted with the following words:

'Tis not oak which here I place
But good fortune—by its grace
May it never pass away
But ever in my dwelling stay!

PURSLANE. Besides protecting the unwary against the assaults of evil spirits, purslane was also thought by the wise to be a sure protection against "blastings by lightning or planets [bad aspects] and burning of gunpowder."

RUE. An ancient and time-honored amulet. The witches of Italy used to sew a sprig of rue, a morsel of bread, a pinch of coarse salt, and a few seeds of cumin into a little bag with red thread and say these words:

This bag I sew for luck to me,
And also to my family;
That it may keep by night and day
Troubles and illness far away!

HERBAL LOVE CHARMS AND DIVINATIONS

Complicated sorcery like that in *The Greater Key of Solomon* with its fancy incenses, silken cloths, and attention to fine astrological detail was useful to only the wealthier and more leisured practitioner of the black arts. The village wizard and wise woman would be far more likely to make use of lesser grimoires, like the *Black Hen*, watered-down versions of *Solomon* with less exacting ritual demands. Rudimentary charm books, such as nineteenth-century *Egyptian Secrets of Albertus Magnus* and *Long Lost Friend* (which incidentally, are still on sale), might also be their Bible. Within the pages of these books may be found a mixture of the same old traditional Saxon, Teutonic, and Celtic beliefs blended with much herbal lore and sometimes the Hebraic magic of *Solomon*, but Christianized throughout and peppered with invocations to Jesus, the Holy Trinity and the Virgin Mary. Most of the spells and potions are addressed to matters which concern country folk most: curing disease in the home as well as in the barn, protection from fire, theft, pests, and so on. Blood-stopping spells occur frequently, and so do antiwart charms.

Similar in style and content to charm books were many of the old dream books, little fortunetelling volumes usually ascribed to the authorship of "Mother So-and-So." Besides giving rules for telling fortunes by cards or palmistry or dreams or any other of the time-honored methods, the pseudonymous authors nearly always include a section on love spells and divinations. Often, for the spell to work, they have to be practiced on the eve of some saint's day, which gives a good indication of their age, for most saints' days are Christianized pagan festivals. Again, as with the traditional love potions of Chapter 5, we see paganism popping up wearing a new hat.

The Ash Tree Spell

To gain a prophetic dream of one's future true love, a sprig of the mystical ash should be plucked with these words:
> Even ash, even ash, I pluck thee,
> This night my true love for to see;
> Neither in his rick or in his rear,
> But in the clothes he does every day wear!

The Hempseed Spell

To cast a spell on one's true love, the prospective bride should sow hempseed either simply in nine furrows or, according to other accounts, on St. Valentine's Eve or Midsummer's Eve around a church as the clock strikes midnight.
> Hempseed I sow, hempseed I sow,
> The young man that I love
> Come after me, and mow.
> I sow; I sow;
> Then my own dear
> Come here, come here:
> And mow; and mow!

If the nine-furrow method is used, the charm must be repeated nine times, once for each furrow. Otherwise just keep chanting until you finish circling the church. Your true love will look you up the next day. The minister's reaction to the circle of pot that springs up around his church in a week or so will also be worth watching for.

A Poppy Spell

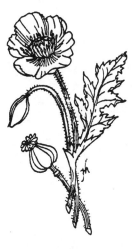

This Italian spell can be adapted to any type of prophetic dream, not merely one concerned with matters of love.

Make a hole in a poppy pod and empty out the seeds. Now fold up a small piece of paper with the question you want answered written on it, insert it in the pod, and place it under your pillow last thing at night, saying these words:

> In the name of heaven, the stars
> and the moon
> May I dream, and that full soon,
> If this I see [name your wish].

WHITE POPPY
(*Papaver somniferum*)

If you dream of your wish, it's sure to come true.

A Willow Spell

Willows were always being used by witches and lovelorn maidens to secure their heart's desires by supernormal means when all other methods had been exhausted. Take a green, pliable willow osier, and tie a firm knot in it, uttering these words as you do:

> This knot I tie,
> This knot I knit,
> For that true love
> Whom I know not yet!

Keep the osier hidden in a safe place until your true love turns up.

A Wormwood Charm

On St. Luke's Day (October 18) take marigold flowers, a sprig of marjoram, thyme, and a little wormwood; dry them before a fire, rub them to powder; then sift it through a fine piece of lawn, and simmer it over a slow fire, adding a small quantity of virgin honey and vinegar. Anoint yourself with this when you go to bed, saying the following lines three times, and you will dream of your partner "that is to be":

St. Luke, St. Luke, be kind to me,
In dreams let me my true love see.

Yarrow Spells

"Bad man's plaything," *Achillea millefolium*, crops up again and again in old love charms. Here are two, the first apparently a variant of the sixteenth-century herb-gathering charm mentioned a few pages back, the second an astrologically derived one which probably indicates a seventeenth- or eighteenth-century origin.

The girl seeking to dream of her future husband or lover should pluck a stalk of yarrow growing from a young man's grave with these words:

Yarrow, sweet yarrow, the first that I have found,
In the name of Jesus Christ, I pluck it from the ground,
As Jesus loved sweet Mary, and took her for his dear,
So in my dream this night, I hope my true love will appear!

The second spell calls for an ounce of regular yarrow (no graveyard plundering here), which should be sewn into a sachet and placed under the pillow. The following charm must be pronounced too:

Thou pretty herb of Venus' tree,
Thy true name it is yarrow;
Now who my bosom friend must be,
Pray tell thou me to-morrow!

HERBS OF ILL OMEN

Witches and cunning-men of the fifteenth and sixteenth centuries were forever conjuring up spirits and ghosts for questioning and making them appear in crystals, magic mirrors, or triangles drawn on the ground. The grimoires and spell-books, such as *The Greater Key of Solomon*, are full of instructions on how to do this. They often required powerful herbal incenses, which gives us a clue to what was really going on. Today's psychologists know a lot more about hallucinations than was known in the sixteenth century. A hallucination can look just as substantial as reality, as any hypnotist will tell you. When a demon did look out of the mirror at the cunning-man or his client, who was to say that it was only a figment of his imagination?

Today we know a bit more about clairvoyance and extrasensory perception, too. Often information received by extrasensory means seems to come to the clairvoyant in symbolic form, so the answers to the questions posed by the fifteenth-century conjurer—generally of the "who stole the silverware" variety—may not always have been so insubstantial as their demon bearers were. Significantly, many of the herbs the conjurer burned as incense while he called upon the spirits contained narcotic or psychoactive drugs, which obviously helped to put him and his clients into a state of semitrance suitable for clairvoyance. Conversely, those herbs he burned to exorcise and banish the demons at the end of the ceremony were often stimulants, like asafoetida, and could well have served to reverse the effects of the narcotic ones.

Here are three typical sorcerer's incenses of a narcotic nature traditionally used in demon conjuring. Unfortunately, no proportions were included in the accounts they are taken from.

Sorcerer's Incense I

Wormwood	Chicory	Camphor
Hemp	Cardamom	Coriander
Flax	Anise	St. John's wort
Lignum aloes		

Sorcerer's Incense II

Reed	Pomegranate skin	Red saunders
Fennel root	Henbane	Black poppy

Sorcerer's Incense III

Coriander	Liquor of black poppy	Sandalwood
Hemlock	Fennel	Henbane
Parsley		

Each of these recipes contains one or more of the three deadly *h*'s of witchcraft: hemp, henbane, and hemlock. All three plants contain extremely powerful narcotic and psychoactive alkaloids. They are very dangerous to play around with, and are on the restricted list of the FDA, so don't be disappointed if you can't find any listed in herb mail-order catalogs. Some Canadian companies do stock some of them, however, but they will not export them, as customs laws regarding illegal drugs (and these are illegal) are very stringent. If you want to try looking for them growing wild, then of course no one can stop you. Be careful what you do with them, though. They're not called witch's herbs for nothing.

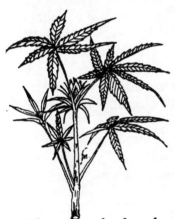

HEMP. *Cannabis sativa* or *indica* hardly needs describing these days. The plant is theoretically an annual, although it can continue to flourish throughout the winter in warmer climates. It generally grows to between three and fifteen feet in height, although higher growths have been recorded. Its serrated leaves are palmate, with between five and seven separate leaflets to each palm, light green and downy on the undersides, darker above. It bears small yellow flowers. Hemp may be found growing wild throughout Asia Minor, Iraq, Iran, northern India, southern Siberia, and some parts of the United States, notably the valleys of the Mississippi and Missouri. Its active principle, cannabinol, is contained within the female flowering tops, and in its pure state produces a state of exhilarating intoxication which may be accompanied by hallucinations; hence its use in sorcery. The crude resin extracted from hemp is known as hashish, an Arabic word from which our word *assassin* derives. The Assassins were a group of eleventh-century Moslem fanatics who, under the direction of their leader Hassan-I-Sabah, the Old Man of the Mountain, were responsible for a series of far-flung political murders and intrigues. Hassan was thought to have gained dominance over his devotees by the clever use of hashish.

Hemp turns up in a lot of old sorcery concoctions. One remarkably to-the-point clairvoyance recipe calls for hemp and mugwort, an herb legendary for its power of conferring second sight.

These plants should be smeared on a polished-steel mirror, and also burned as incense before it for good measure. Visions were said to appear in the mirror if you gazed in it long enough.

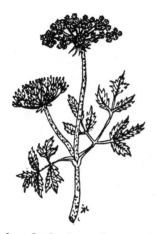

HEMLOCK (*Conium maculatum*). The Greeks of the fourth century B.C. used a hemlock drink as a means of executing condemned criminals. Plato describes the tragic death of his teacher Socrates from such a hemlock cup. Both true hemlock and its close cousin, water hemlock (cowbane or *Cicuta virosa*), grow on damp waste ground and beside streams. The hemlock may be distinguished from the water hemlock and other Umbelliferae by its smooth red-spotted stem and finely divided leaves. Whereas all parts of the hemlock give off a peculiar mousy odor, the water hemlock smells a little like parsley. They're both very, very poisonous, and herbalists generally steer well clear of them. The active principle of the true hemlock is coniine, a volatile narcotic oil whose misuse will produce paralysis and death from asphyxia. Water hemlock contains cicutoxin, which has similar properties.

The Greater Key of Solomon advocates the use of hemlock in the manufacture of the sorcerer's black-handled Knife, the tool with which he traces the magic circle he must stand in when he conjures up demons.

"It should be made ... in the day and hour of Saturn, and dipped in the blood of a black cat and in the juice of hemlock," says the grimoire. "Thou shalt place it thrice in the fire until it become red-hot, and each time thou shalt immerse it in the aforesaid blood and juice ... and upon the hilt thou shalt write with the pen of Art, commencing from the point and going towards the hilt [these] ... Characters and Names ... Which being completed, thou shalt wrap it in a black silk cloth."

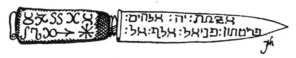

KING SOLOMON'S BLACK-HANDLED KNIFE

This barbarous use of blood to temper a blade, from a historical point of view, is not so strange as it sounds. It was a common practice during the Middle Ages. The blades of Toledo were said to be so tempered; the long-recognized property of blood to harden red-hot iron into steel is due to its high nitrogen content. The poor black cat, like the hemlock itself, was thought to be an animal "ruled" by Saturn, the planet that lent its dark power to the knife to "strike terror and fear into the spirits," a very ancient shamanistic practice.

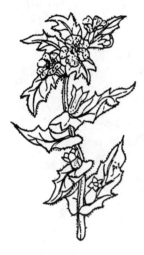

HENBANE
(Hyoscyamus niger)

HENBANE (*Hyoscyamus niger*). Pleasant in neither appearance nor odor, this "cursed hebenon" as Shakespeare refers to it in *Hamlet*, grows in waste, sandy ground with thick, rounded hairy stems, pale-green downy leaves, and dull-yellow flowers with purple stripes. All parts exude a pungent odor, and are extremely poisonous. The drugs hyoscine and hyoscymine are derived from henbane, and this may partially explain its use as an ingredient in so-called witches' sabbat ointments of the sixteenth and seventeenth centuries. Johannes Baptista Porta, an occult philosopher of the sixteenth century, was the first person to record actual recipes for this unguent.[20] Witches were supposed to anoint themselves and their broomsticks with it before flying off to their nocturnal revels:

[20] *Magia Naturalis*, 1560.

TRADITIONAL WITCHES' OINTMENTS

Recipe I

ELEOSELINUM. This is the "heleioselinum" of Dioscorides, what today is called *Apium graveolens* or smallage by herbalists. It is used as a tonic and combined with damiana or coca to make a rheumatism remedy.

ACONITE. A very dangerous herb once used to poison wolf-traps, hence its old name wolfbane. Herbalists use it externally in lumbago and rheumatism rubs.

POPLAR FRONDS. Today balm of Gilead, as poplar buds are called, is used by herbalists to make a soothing application for external bruises and abrasions.

SOOT. Dioscorides tells us that soot should be used on open sores and ulcers to form a scab.

Recipe II

SIUM. Probably smallage, although some writers have conjectured that this could be water hemlock. Conium, the latter's close relative was used by the Greeks and Arabs in rubs to cure painful joints and skin conditions.

Acorum vulgaris. This is the "acoron" of Dioscorides, *Acorus calamus* or sweet flag today, an herb not introduced generally to Europe until 1574, when Clusius, a Viennese botanist, succeeded in growing a slip brought from the Tartars in Asia Minor in his garden. When Porta wrote of it, it was obviously quite a rare ingredient.

CINQUEFOIL. Herbalists use this externally as an astringent lotion for abrasions and scratches.

BAT'S BLOOD. Either a ritual ingredient or a figment of Porta's imagination. Bat's blood is referred to in *The Greater Key of Solomon,* so it did have a precedent.

Solanum somniferum. "Sleep-bearing solanum" is undoubtedly *Atropa belladonna,* deadly nightshade, a plant from which the drug belladonna is extracted. Used externally it numbs the skin like novocaine. It is used in herbal sciatica and gout preparations.

OIL. Pork lard is generally used by the old herbalists, although sensation-minded demonologists such as Montague Summers have construed this to be baby's fat!

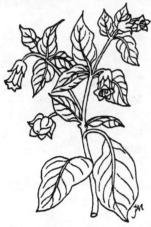

DEADLY NIGHTSHADE
(*Atropa belladonna*)

The general opinion over the past twenty years has been that the ointments were themselves hallucinogenic, thus accounting for the fantastic descriptions of the sabbat that witches gave. Aconite, water hemlock, calamus (in quantity), and deadly nightshade would be hallucinogenic if not fatal when taken internally. However, on closer examination it is difficult to see how these ingredients applied externally in ointment form could have been, even if, as some writers postulate, the scabrous condition of the witch's skin permitted a certain amount of the drug to enter her bloodstream. But the ointments *would* have had the effect of making the skin insensible to superficial pain and cold and maybe even given the naked witch the feeling that she was in some way suspended above the ground, the traditional "flying" phenomenon. The use of calamus at this early date is also interesting for it points to a Middle Eastern derivation of the recipe. Certainly the sabbat, the ecstatic revel of medieval witchery, sounds more like an Asian shamanic seance, a Thracian bacchanal, or the North African circle of whirling dervishes than anything indigenous to Europe.

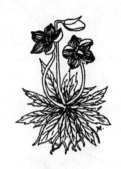

BLACK HELLEBORE
(*Helleborus niger*)

So these then are the three dangerous *h*'s of witchcraft. Actually there is a fourth, hellebore, a plant whose poisonous root is mentioned by Francis Barrett as an incense ingredient of the planet Mars. However, there are also less illegal and just as traditional recipes for achieving witchy results in case you feel like experimenting. Here are four of them.

Scrying Incenses

Scrying is the old name witches used for divination by staring into a mirror, a crystal, or even a glass of water and waiting for pictures to form in the mind's eye. We call it clairvoyance today. Any one of these incenses could be burned in front of your mirror or crystal while you scried. Tisanes composed of wormwood or fraxinella were also thought to help.

1. Linseed and psellium.
2. Violet roots and wild parsley.
3. Anise seed and camphor.
4. Powdered valerian root, saffron, wormwood, St. John's wort juice.
5. Wormwood.
6. Dittany of Crete.

Numbers 3, 5, and 6 are the only ones that smell remotely reasonable as incenses. The rest are rather foul. As to their legendary powers, you'll have to try them for yourselves. Maybe they'll work for you if you have the talent.

Witches are rumored to have learned much of their herbal lore from elves, those mysterious "good folk" believed by the European peasantry to inhabit barrows and burial mounds of bygone peoples, emerging only on ancient pagan festivals like Halloween and Midsummer. Who or what elves, or fairies, as they were known to the Celts, were has been a matter of considerable debate among folklorists. Maybe they were folk memories of rustic pagan deities. That was Jakob Grimm's view. W. Y. Evans-Wentz thought that they were the spirits of the ancient dead. Margaret Murray, on the other hand, suggested that they were real people, bands of "heathens," people of the heath, remnants of the pre-Christian population who elected to live apart from the Christian community and pursue their own ways. Bessie Dunlop, a sixteenth-century Scottish witch, claimed to have received her magic craft from them. Joan of Arc was thought to have consorted with them; and the Reverend Robert Kirk, a respected seventeenth-century Scottish minister, claimed he had had the gift of clairvoyance bestowed upon him by them.

To finish this chapter, here are two quaint herbal ointments that were supposed to open and close the doors to the elfin king-doms to the witch. The first is taken from an early-seventeenth-century manuscript; the second, an anti-elf concoction, from the tenth-century *Leech-book of Bald and Cild*. You will undoubtedly recognize a number of old witch favorites among the ingredients of the latter.

A Salve to Enable One to See the Fairies [21]

[Take] A pint of sallet oyle and put it into a vial glasse; and first wash it with rose-water and marygolde water; the flowers to be gathered towards the east. Wash it till the oyle becomes white, then put into the glasse, and then put thereto the budds of hollyhocke, the flowers of marygolde, the flowers or toppes of wild thyme the budds of young hazle, and the thyme must be gathered near the side of a hill where fairies used to be; and take the grasse of a fairy throne; then all these put into the oyle in the glasse and sette it to dissolve three days in the sunne and then keep it for thy use.

A Salve against the elfin race and nocturnal visitors, and for women with whom the devil hath carnal commerce [22]

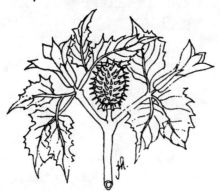

THORNAPPLE (*Datura stramonium*), also known to witches as devil's apple

Take the Ewe Hop plant, Wormwood, Bishopswort, Lupin, Ashthroat, Henbane, Harewort, Viper's bugloss, Heatherberry plants, Cropleek, Garlic, Grains of Hedgerife, Githrife, and Fennel. These herbs are to be put in a vessel and placed beneath the altar where nine masses are sung over them. They should then be boiled in butter and mutton fat and much

---

[21] From a manuscript dated 1600 in the Ashmolean Museum at Oxford.
[22] From the *Leech-book of Bald and Cild*.

holy salt added; the salve should then be strained through a cloth; and what remains of the worts thrown into running water. The victim's forehead and eyes are to be anointed with the ointment, and he should be censed with incense and signed often with the sign of the cross!

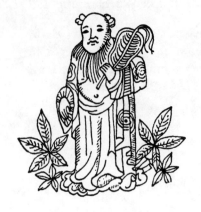

7

HERBAL IMMORTALITY: ELIXIRS OF LIFE

"AND THE LORD GOD SAID, Behold, the man is become as one of us, to know good and evil: and now, lest he put forth his hand, and take also of the tree of life, and eat, and live for ever: Therefore the Lord God sent him forth from the garden of Eden, to till the ground from whence he was taken. So he drove out the man; and he placed at the east of the garden of Eden cherubims, and a flaming sword which turned every way, to keep the way of the tree of life."

The Bible is not alone in vesting the secret of immortality in a plant. Most of the ancient civilizations of the world have myths concerning a tree or herb which confers deathlessness upon the possessor. The Babylonians believed the herb grew at the bottom of the ocean. The Persians believed it was a tree planted on Mount Harait by the great God of Light, Ahura Mazda himself. The Greeks thought it was an apple tree, and placed it in the Garden of the Hesperides, a remote island guarded by dragons; and the *Mahabharata*, an ancient text of the Hindus, mentions a paradisal plant from which an elixir of life known as *soma* was brewed. The Celtic Druids imagined that the mistletoe, that mysterious golden bough which flourishes upon oak and ash and thorn, being in some way bound up with the ever-living sun itself, contained the secrets of life in its berry.

It was in China, however, that the search for longevity stepped out of the pages of mythology and became a historically documented pursuit. Most herbal longevity lore is derived from these Chinese sources. Closely associated with the practice of Taoism, the religion introduced by the philosopher Lao-tze around 560 B.C., the search for the elixir of life became a common theme in Chinese alchemy. As Arabic alchemists like Razi postulated ten centuries later, the Philosopher's Stone, that hypothetical substance which hastened the evolution of base metals and turned them into silver and gold, was also thought by the Chinese to prolong life indefinitely. However, whereas the Arabs turned solely to the realm of minerals and metallic ores for their search, the early Chinese alchemists flung their net wide to include the entire vegetable kingdom too. Chung-li Ch'uan, one of the Eight Immortals, legendary patron saints of Taoism, was said to have lived from 1112 B.C. to 249 B.C. by means of such an elixir. The *Lieh Hsien Ch'uan*, an eighth-century B.C. collection of biographies of these Immortals, suspected the pine, the cypress, and the peach of containing the drug of longevity in their leaves. Ko-hung, an alchemist who wrote under the pseudonym Pao P'u-tsu (literally "the Master who preserves his pristine simplicity"), embellished these beliefs, claiming that the man who fed on powdered cypress nuts might live to be a thousand years old. In addition, the *Lieh Hsien Ch'uan* singles out the leek, cinnamon, shepherd's-purse seeds, angelica, and sunflower as life prolongers. Other seekers after immortality placed coriander seeds and chervil on the list.

But by far the most prestigious Oriental longevity herbs were *Hydrocotyle asiatica minor*, known in India as *gotu kola*, in China as *fo-ti-tieng*, and most important of all the time-honored ginseng, named by the Emperor Shen-nung "King of All Herbs."

Ginseng

AMERICAN GINSENG
(Panax quinquefolium)

The name Ginseng is derived from the Chinese *jen shen*, which has been variously translated as "wonder of the world root" and "man-plant." It owes its last name to its extraordinary root, which is forked like the fabled mandrake of the West, and frequently grows into a doll-like shape. One of the American Indian names for ginseng is *Garantoquen*, which is said to mean much the same thing. The herb also appears in American herbals as five fingers, tartar root, ninsin, red berry, Chinese seng, and man's health. Incidentally, true ginseng should not be confused with blue cohosh (*Caulophyllum thalictroides*), which sometimes goes by the names yellow ginseng and blue ginseng. "Red" ginseng, on the other hand, often touted for its power as a fine stimulant, is regular ginseng root that has been macerated in a blend of other herbal extracts; these give it its uncharacteristic color. The uplift to be gained from red ginseng is due to the presence of kola nuts in the herbal blend.

Panax ginseng or *shinseng*, to give it its correct botanical title, was first advocated by the Chinese emperor Shen-nung five thousand years ago. It was, he said, a tonic which prolonged life and ministered to man at all levels of his being: body, mind, and spirit. The *Atharva Veda*, one of the sacred books of the Aryans who invaded India from the area now called Iran between 3000 and 1500 B.C., also extols ginseng's virtues as an aphrodisiac and sexual rejuvenator. Apparently the use of ginseng was as widespread in the Far East as it was ancient. One of the last herbs to officially come West, ginseng did not attract the notice of Europeans until the early eighteenth century. A French missionary observed that the Chinese among whom he worked held one particular plant in veneration. Its roots were considered so valuable that the emperor regarded them as his own special property, and the major portion of the revenue derived from their sale had to be paid into the imperial coffers. Father Jartoux also noted that Chinese doctors used this plant as a major ingredient in all their more potent medicines. He states in his account that this "ginseng" herb was used to combat fatigue, tumors, and even the ravages of old age. Jartoux saw no reason to disbelieve these claims, for he himself had experienced the relief a dose of the herb provided from bodily exhaustion after a long journey.

However, it was not until 1718, when another French missionary, this time a Jesuit working in Canada, first tentatively identified the American *Panax quinquefolius* with the Chinese *Panax ginseng,* and had his suspicions confirmed by botanists in Paris, that the ginseng truly became a concern of Western herbalists. In the same year, the Jesuits began employing American Indians to comb the forests of the north for the herb, not as one might think, for Western pharmacists, but to sell to China. The Indians the Jesuits employed knew the herb well enough: they had employed it for centuries in love potions.

By 1748 the price of ginseng shipped to Canton had reached $1 per pound. Twenty-eight years later it had risen to $1.17. It was an obvious sure-fire investment. In 1895 the Great Ginseng Boom hit the United States. Natural supplies of the herb were running low, and ginseng farms had sprung up in the meantime to meet the need. Inflated claims about the fortunes to be made from ginseng farming prompted wild speculation and investment; but the bubble burst in 1904 when a leaf disease struck the American farms and ruined the major portion of the crop—a disaster considering the fact that a ginseng plant takes from five to seven years to mature. The disaster, of course, drove the price up: by 1912 it had risen to $7.20 a pound, and during the next fifty years it more than doubled. Today (in 1973) it retails at between $45 and $65 a pound, or around $5 an ounce.

302 / MASTERING HERBALISM

There are several different types of ginseng on the market. The wild variety, allegedly more potent than the cultivated plant, is practically unobtainable today and sells at a considerably higher price. And of the two varieties, Korean *Panax ginseng* (also known as Chinese or Asiatic ginseng) and American *Panax quinquefolius*, the Chinese is more desirable. There is also a Japanese variety, but ginseng aficionados don't think much of it. So ideally the best type of ginseng one can buy is wild Korean, and the most undistinguished variety is cultivated Japanese or American; but then there aren't that many herbalists who can really tell the difference. In fact, I have heard it rumored that the roots imported to the Orient from the States are often simply relabeled and sold back again at a profit, and no one is any the wiser.

HOW TO USE IT. Before embarking on instructions on how to grow your own—you'll need the patience of Job if you intend to do this—we should take a look at some of the ways herbalists use ginseng. Western usage to a large degree parallels that of the Chinese, whose practices have in many ways come down unchanged from Shen-nung's day. Even the shift in political climate has done little to change the basic "medicine of the land." The stern injunction against using metal of any sort to prepare ginseng (except, on occasion, silver) reflects the antiquity of the tradition. Bowls and implements of wood, pottery, glass, or enamel must be used instead.

CHINESE GINSENG PRESCRIPTIONS

To Extract Ginseng Essence

Boil powdered ginseng root in water until only a thick sediment remains. Strain and bottle, but use soon. Powdered ginseng root may also be steeped in five times its weight in alcohol to produce a tincture. (Commercially produced condensed Korean ginseng extract comes in a pretty little white jar and smells a bit like beef extract. A dilute variety mixed with honey and spices is also available.)

Ginseng Digestive

Mix powdered ginseng root with the white of an egg. Take three times daily.

Ginseng Sedative

Take either a light soup of ginseng root and bamboo shoots or a decoction of equal parts of ginseng root and dried orange peel flavored with honey before going to bed at night.

Ginseng to Stimulate the Circulation

Drink 1 cup per day of ginseng essence (the diluted extract) mixed with honey and cinnamon.

Ginseng Diaphoretic

One liang (36 grams) ginseng should be boiled in 2 cups water until the liquid has reduced by half. The resultant liquid should be diluted with pure spring water before being taken.

Ginseng Sexual Restorative

Boil green ginseng with orange peel, and mix in a little ginseng essence.

General Ginseng Tonic

Boil raw, expressed ginseng juice, honey, and ginseng root down into a thick glue. When it has hardened, cut it into nut-sized nuggets. Dissolve one of these in a cup of hot rice water per dose.

THE RECOGNIZED EFFECTS OF GINSENG

About as far as the more cautious Western herbalists will go regarding the uses of the *Panax* (the plant figures in neither the American nor the British pharmacopoeias today) is to say that it is

304 / MASTERING HERBALISM

a mild digestive stimulant. However, this is not to say that the root is scorned in the West—far from it. There exists a considerable literature upon the subject. A number of doctors and herbalists both in the United States and in Europe have tested the herb and come up with a list of properties and principles that are as yet unrecognized by orthodox medicine. It is only fair to add that "orthodoxy" has not remained silent, either, and there have been a bevy of rebuttals too. The FDA casts a very disapproving eye on any company claiming medical miracles from ginseng. It is a controversy which, like the question of herbal medicine in general, still rages on. But like the entire art of herbalism, the use of ginseng has five thousand years of history behind it. The Chinese are a remarkably long-lived people, and present-day science is constantly revising its tenets; so who can honestly say that five thousand years of unshaken belief is not worth a little personal investigation? For my part I can only say that I don't care what "authority" says. From my own experience I have found ginseng to be a remarkable herb, as invigorating as it is healthful. As to whether I shall live to a ripe old 123 like Shen-nung, only time can tell. But I'm game to giving it a try. Many people concur in the opinion that ginseng at the very least seems to act as a general all-around tonic—not necessarily a cure-all as *Panax* would imply, but rather a maintainer of health. Among the many conditions ginseng has been said to help, the following extraordinarily varied and sometimes contradictory examples can be mentioned. How many of them are bona fide and how many are wishful thinking remains to be seen. However, the news that the USSR seized the entire crop of North Korean ginseng during the nineteen-fifties and is now engaged in vigorously farming the herb for itself in southern Siberia leads one to suspect that we are not the only people who are becoming aware of the potentialities of this mysterious herb.

CONDITIONS PURPORTEDLY ALLEVIATED BY GINSENG

Aging (ginseng is thought to slow down cell degeneration)
Arthritis
Biliousness
Bladder complaints
Circulatory problems
Constipation
Depression
Diarrhea
Drug addition
Exhaustion
Forgetfulness
Frigidity
Gout
Hepatitis after-effects
Heart palpitations
High blood pressure
Impotence
Indigestion
Insomnia
Itching
Kidney complaints
Loss of appetite
Low blood pressure
Nausea
Nervous exhaustion
Neuritis
Postoperative effects
Premature loss of hair
Rheumatism
Sciatica
Skin rashes
Throat complaints

CONSTITUENTS OF GINSENG

So far the chemical analysis of ginseng has proved surprisingly unsensational. No mysterious vitamin X has yet shown up to explain the herb's extraordinary powers. It may well be that the key to them lies in the plant's individual combination of chemical elements. These are thought to include starch; mucilage; resin; the glucoside saponin; a small amount of essential oil; panacon, an element peculiar to ginseng (maybe this is it?); vitamins B_1 and B_2; sulphur salts of phosphorus, aluminum, iron, manganese, cobalt, and copper; and various enzymes, like amylase.

HOW TO USE GINSENG

The redoubtable Mrs. Grieve blithely prescribed that a decoction of an entire ½ ounce of ginseng root be downed as a tea or soup every morning. At around $2.50 a throw this seems a bit extravagant to today's herbal enthusiast, who tends rather to employ one of the following, more economical, methods:

1. A tea made from a few slices of the root, simmered in 1 cup water in a covered enamel or Pyrex pot or double boiler for 1 to 4 hours. Three tablespoons to be taken during or before meals.

2. A little powdered ginseng root sprinkled on vegetable juices, salads, meat, fish, soup, or cereals.

3. Powdered ginseng root taken with meals in gelatin capsules. Most health-food stores and many pharmacies now stock these. The usual dosage seems to be around 8 or 9 grains of powdered ginseng per capsule.

4. Ginseng tea made from ½ teaspoon of the leaves, flowers, or powdered root in 1 cup hot water.

5. Ginseng tincture. Steep the leaves or powdered root in a tightly covered screw-top jar with equal parts of potable alcohol and water. The ginseng should be barely covered by the liquid. Leave it to macerate for 2 weeks before straining off the tincture. The tincture may be mixed with honey, maple syrup, or molasses. An adult dose is between 10 and 15 minims (drops) daily.

6. Simply chew on a piece of the root. This is the way Chinese peasants used it.

7. Ginseng leaves and flowers smoked as a tobacco. I can't vouch for the effectiveness of this, but many people are doing it nowadays.

GROWING YOUR OWN GINSENG

Panax quinquefolium, American ginseng, comes from the same plant family as the sarsaparilla and the garden aralia. It grows wild in cool, shaded, wooded areas throughout Canada and the central and eastern United States. So if you plan on growing your own you must give your crop plenty of shade during the summer months, but make sure it has plenty of air circulation around it too. A framework hut of wood laths is about the best way of providing this. Your wood strips should run in a north-south direction. Don't use fine nylon mesh or burlap on the frame, however, as these interfere with the air circulation. If you have a shady garden or a small wood or spinney near you, then you have no problem. The plants may be grown from seed, seedlings, or root stocks, and they need a rich, loamy soil like that found in the maple and oak forests of the northern states. The soil should be well drained and fairly light. Too sandy a soil is said to produce tough, flinty roots. Ginseng can be grown in pots easily enough, but if you plan on laying out a seed bed dig up the soil to a depth of at least 6 inches and be sure to remove any weeds and rootlets from neighboring trees. Then mix into the natural soil an equal amount of fiber-free woodland soil and enough sand to prevent the mixture from hardening into cakes after you water. If you are planting seedlings, on the other hand, you'll have to dig the bed down to a depth of 8 inches. Roots need at least 12 inches. Cover the plants with a forest-leaf, cornstalk, or buckwheat-straw mulch during frosty winter months, but again, make sure the mulch contains no weeds. Woodland soil or rotted hickory or basswood sawdust mixed with bone meal may be mixed in as fertilizer at a ratio of 1 pound per square yard. If you plan to leave the seeds where they are to grow to mature plants, give them 8 inches' separation from one another. The seeds themselves should be planted at a depth of 1 inch. If you take them directly from a parent plant in the fall, don't allow them to dry out, but plant them immediately and mulch them well. They'll begin sprouting the following spring.

Seedlings, though more expensive, yield a ginseng crop sooner than seeds. For ginseng—and here's the rub, I'm afraid—requires between five and seven years to mature from seed. The quickest method of growing it, therefore, is from young roots, which can be planted anytime between October and April. They should be set at a depth of 2 inches, allowing 8 inches between plants. A young root of this sort will yield a crop in about three or four years. If you plan to farm ginseng on a regular basis, five beds containing seeds, one-, two-, and three-year-old seedlings, and roots will yield continuous crops beginning three or four years after planting. After harvesting the matured ginseng plants grown from the roots, the seeds from the other plants should be grown in the now empty bed. This will ensure you a continuous annual harvest.

HARVESTING YOUR GINSENG

Ginseng leaves may be harvested at any time of the year. Mature ginseng roots should be dug up in their fifth to seventh year around mid-October. A reasonable specimen ought to measure at least 4 inches long, 1 inch thick below the top, and weigh around 1 ounce. The older the root the better, however, both from the herbal and the marketing point of view. Undersize roots can easily be replanted for an additional few months if necessary. When uprooting them be careful not to injure them with your digging tool. If you want to adhere to the oldest Chinese practices, it should not be an iron one. A wooden stick is quite adequate in most cases if your soil has been kept in good condition.

Carefully rinse the soil from the roots, taking care not to snap off their forks or scrape off any of their characteristic rings. They should then be dried on a wire lattice [1] in a well-ventilated, heated room. Either start drying them between 60° to 80° F. and increase the temperature to 90° after a couple of days, or begin at 100° to 110° and reduce the temperature to 90° once the roots have wilted. The larger 2-inch-diameter roots will take about 6 weeks to dry, the smaller ones less. Once brittle, they should be stored in a dry, airy, and rodent-proof place until you need to use them.[2]

[1] See Chapter 8.

[2] For further information see United States Department of Agriculture "Farmer's Bulletin" No. 2201, available from the Superintendent of Documents, U.S. Government Printing Office, Washington, D.C. 20402.

Gotu Kola and Fo-ti-tieng

Hydrocotyle vulgaris, or common pennywort, is mentioned by both Gerard and Culpeper with conflicting degrees of enthusiasm about what was then its customary use, a diuretic and specific for gallstones. Culpeper approved of it, but Gerard disapproved, chiefly on account of its penchant for producing footrot in sheep. But neither of them knew about its exotic cousin, *Hydrocotyle asiatica minor,* flourishing on the other side of the globe in South Africa and India.

The December 22, 1932, edition of the *Ceylon Daily News* carried a story about a wonder herb new to Western eyes, called gotu kola. The article aroused a great deal of interest, for it claimed that the plant had been used by the Indians and Sinhalese down the centuries, and hailed it as the Secret of Perpetual Youth. It went on to detail how the leaves were discovered to have, among other salutory effects, an energizing and preservative action upon the brain cells of the taker. "Two leaves a day will keep old age away" was quoted as an old Sinhalese proverb, which admittedly sounds like a journalist's version of "an apple a day keeps the doctor away."

The following year, however, *The New York Times* came up with an even more amazing story of a certain recently deceased professor Li-chung Yun. The professor's age, as far as could be ascertained, was not a mere 123 years like the legendary Shen-nung, but a staggering 256! A researcher at the Minkue University later investigated this prodigy, and confirmed the fact that Li had indeed been born in 1677. It was also noted that Li-chung Yun was living with his twenty-fourth wife at the time of his demise, and far from presenting the appearance of someone in the last throes of senility, had retained the look of a fifty-year-old man until the time of his death.

The secret to which Li attributed his longevity was an herb he used, not ginseng—although he used that regularly too—but a certain *fo-ti-tieng,* which unhelpfully translated as Elixir of Long Life. P. de Layman, a director of the Herbal Institute of London, did

310 / MASTERING HERBALISM

some research on this enigmatic herb, and finally identified it as none other than *Hydrocotyle asiatica minor*, gotu kola.

Today *Hydrocotyle asiatica minor* is almost as popular a runner as ginseng in the longevity stakes. There remains a certain amount of confusion among herbalists about its correct name, however, chiefly on account of the fact that a commercial company copyrighted the name fo-ti-tieng for its own herbal formula some time ago, and is now very indignant about seeing simple *Hydrocotyle asiatica minor* advertised by that title. Harvest Health, Inc., a mail-order herb-supply store in Michigan, claims the registered fo-ti-tieng formula contains *Hydrocotyle asiatica minor*; meadow-sweet, rich in salts and vitamin C; and kola nuts, which, in addition to manifesting the same properties as caffeine, are considered by some herbalists a good all-around tonic.

THE CONSTITUENTS OF HYDROCOTYLE ASIATICA MINOR

As far as we know, *Hydrocotyle* contains chiefly tannin and an essential oil, vellarin. The taste and smell of the oil is bitter and pungent, but not so objectionable as to prevent the herb's being eaten in the East with rice or bread.

PROPERTIES

The conservative view of *Hydrocotyle asiatica minor*'s uses is limited to its applications as an aperient and alternative tonic, although Grieve acknowledges it as a noted remedy for rheumatism, leprosy, and ichthyosis and a poultice for syphilitic ulcers. She does add, however, that whereas small doses have a stimulating effect, large doses act as a narcotic, producing stupor, headache, and possibly even coma. Other herbalists claim that *Hydrocotyle* aids the healing of abscesses, bruises, fevers, neuritis, and even elephantiasis. According to one account, the body should also be exposed to sunlight to ensure maximum effect. But the herb's main attraction, of course, lies in its beguiling promise of longevity through cell rejuvenation. And, as in the case of ginseng, who knows for certain that the cloud of witnesses and centuries of time-honored tradition are wrong? Digitalis was, after all, first discovered in the herbal formula of a Shropshire witch, hardly a respectable place for a scientist to search for a wonder drug. Snakeroot *(Rauwolfia)*, another herb used for centuries in Asia as a sedative, was ultimately discovered by tardy Western scientists to contain the drug reserpine, one of the most valuable tools in the treatment of psychosis since 1952. These are only two examples out of many. Obviously the point to be drawn is that humble herbs should not be scoffed at out of hand but rather deserve every possible consideration as a source of potential curative agents.

EUROPEAN METHODS OF USING HYDROCOTYLE

Hydrocotyle may be infused as a tea, taken powdered in capsule form, or sprinkled upon salads or other foods. It retails in the United States at the time of writing (1973) at between $2 and $6.50 per pound. The infusion dosage advocated is usually 1 teaspoon of the regular dried herb to 1 cup boiling water, taken once a day. I usually add a little honey, cinnamon, and clove to make it more palatable. The powdered herb may also be obtained loose or in capsules, generally size #0, containing about 8 grains of *Hydrocotyle* each.

Other Traditional Longevity Herbs

If you're interested in trying out any of the other herbs rumored by lore and legend to possess life-prolonging and brain-cell-rejuvenating properties, here is a short list of some of the more edible ones.

BALM

Llewelyn, a Prince of Wales, was reported to have lived to the age of 108 by reason of the balm tea he drank in the morning and evening. A certain John Hussey of Sydenham also claimed that balm contained the secret of longevity. He drank balm tea with honey every morning for breakfast, and lived to be 116 years old!

GARLIC

Credited with life-prolonging powers by the inhabitants of the Caucasus, the garlic root may be safely taken in capsule form by those considerate of the feelings of their mates or business associates. Herbal retailers often stock these capsules containing the garlic either powdered or as a concentrated oil. They're also said to improve your memory and mental capacity.

MUGWORT (Artemisia vulgaris)

> If they wad drink nettles in March
> And eat muggons in May,
> Sae mony braw maidens
> Wadna gang to the clay!

scolded a mermaid in the Firth of Clyde as she watched the funeral procession of one such young maiden pass by. Or so they say in Scotland. The legend illustrates the long-held belief that muggons—mugwort—contains life-prolonging tonic qualities.

ROSEMARY

Its traditionally ascribed powers as a brain-stimulant and improver of memory have led some present-day herbalists to speculate on its potentialities as a cell-regenerator.

SAGE

The Chinese said, "Sage for old age," the Romans said, *"Cur moriatur homo cui salvia crescit in horto?"* and the English said, "He that would live for aye, Must eat sage in May." John Evelyn wrote in 1699: " 'Tis a plant, indeed, with so many and wonderful properties as that the assiduous use of it is said to render men immortal."

YERBA MATE *(Ilex paraguayensis)*

Like regular tea and coffee, yerba maté contains both tannin and caffeine, and has a powerful stimulant action. It also contains salts of magnesium, iron, calcium, manganese, silica, and phosphates. A shrub native to South America and a member of the holly family, it is also known by herbalists as Paraguay tea, missionaries' tea, and Jesuits' tea. The celebrated longevity of many of the Argentinian gauchos has been thought to be directly related to their ingestion of maté in quantity. Traditionally the tea should be flavored with burned sugar and lemon, and sucked through a silver tube from a hollow gourd.

Finally, here are two rather wild, not to say impractical, recipes for elixirs of life which have long haunted the pages of herbals. I need hardly add that I include them here for curiosity's sake only.

The first, a breathless, unpunctuated recipe, was recorded by a Dr. Peter Dumoulin of Canterbury in the year 1682; the second is ascribed to the wily sixteenth-century German wizard Abbot Trithemius.

Dr. Dumoulin's Surrup for the Preservation of Long Life [3]

To be done in the Moone of May. Take of the juice of mercury [*Chenopodium Bonus Henricus*] eight pound of the juice of Burridg [borage] two pounds of the juice of Buglosse [alkanet] two pounds mingle these with twelve pounds of Clarrified Honey the whitest you can gett let them boyle together a boyling and pass through a Hippocras Bag of New flannell Infuse in three pints of white wine a quarter of a pound of gentian root and a half a pound of Iris [orris] root or blew Flower de Lis [*Iris pseudacorus*] let them be infused twenty-four houers then strain without squeezing. Put the liquor to that of the herbs and hony boyle them well together to the consistance of a surrup you must order the matter so that one thing stays not for the other but that all be ready together.

A spoonfull of this surrup is to be taken every Morning Fasting.

By way of introduction the manuscript claims that the syrup preserved the life of its inventor, an "Old Gentleman" from "Barbary," for 132 years! Not bad for a cordial.

Abbot Trithemius' Elixir of Longevity
(translated from the Latin)

Take and powder 15 grams of:

Calamus	Anise
Gentian	Caraway seeds
Cinnamon	Amece
Mountain willow	[I haven't been able
(white willow is sometimes used	to translate this]
for general debility of the	Parsley seeds
digestive tract)	Lavender flowers
	Red coral [!]

[3] From Thomas Newington's *M. S. Book of Receipts* (1719).

And add 27 grams of:

Powdered, unpierced pearls [!!]	Bittersweet herb
	Senna leaves
White ginger	Burnt tartar

And lastly 7 grams of:

Mace	Cubebs

Trithemius advocated taking 5 grams of this powder each night for one month, 5 grams in the morning only for the second month, and thereafter 5 grams three times a week. The benefits to be obtained from this dubious brew were "a good stomach, a strong mind, and a tenacious memory." While not recommending that anyone actually try out the worthy abbot's concoction, it is interesting to note that both senna and bittersweet possess strongly diuretic properties, while senna was also frequently prescribed by herbalists in combination with cream of tartar and ginger or cinnamon as a cathartic. So were gentian and senna.

So it begins to look suspiciously as if the secret potion hiding behind Trithemius' cryptic Latin, his secret of "a strong mind and a tenacious memory," was really nothing more than a mighty laxative. Well, *in corpore sano,* they say.

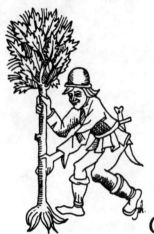

8

GROWING YOUR OWN

OUTDOOR HERB GARDENS

One of the most enjoyable things about growing your own herbs as distinct from showy garden blooms is the relatively low number of do's and dont's you have to concern yourself with. Apart from a few minor and fairly obvious considerations, herbs generally take care of themselves with a minimum of participation from you.

About the most important point to remember is that the majority of the essential oil-bearing herbs like sage, thyme, rosemary, and marjoram originated in the sunny Mediterranean areas, where the soil is stony and not particularly rich. Therefore the ideal herb garden should have a sheltered, sunny location with a medium-light soil. Heavy clay soils should be lightened with topsoil and, if you live in a cold climate, dug up in the fall so that the winter frosts can get at the clay and break it up. Herb growers in colder climates should also arrange to have some sort of protecting windbreak on the north and east sides, ideally a solid fence or wall. If trees or hedges form your screen, make sure you don't plant your herbs too close to them or the tree rootlets will strangle them. The ideal herb garden—the one that takes care of itself to the fullest extent—should be provided with an area of ground lying lower than the rest so that moisture-loving herbs like the mints and angelica can be planted in these damper, low-lying spots. (Failing that, simply give them more water than the other herbs.) You should also arrange to give the mints in particular a good dose of fertilizer in the spring. Any of the commercially available ones will do. If you wish to raise annual herbs such as anise, basil, chervil, coriander, cumin, dill, parsley, and marigold from seed, they are best sown in pots or boxes first, then separated and transferred to your garden or patch later in the spring or early summer. That way you can keep a close eye on predatory slugs and avoid clawing up the young seedlings when you weed your garden. Also, any lengthy watering or hosing you give your herb garden won't beat them flat.

The easiest way to raise herbs is from the seedlings obtainable from most nurseries and many plant stores. Those herbs you cannot find can be obtained by mail from the appropriate mail-order companies listed in the next chapter.

YOUR HERB GARDEN LAYOUT

In the old days paradise gardens were laid out in symmetrical and meaningful patterns. They were designed as mandalas, diagrams drawn with living plants upon the ground, which illustrated symbolically cosmic balance and harmony, the crystallization of divine order out of chaos. This is what the name "paradise garden" implied. Paradise, or Eden, was the grand blueprint of all herb gardens in the old herbalists' eyes, a garden in which every plant ministered to unfallen mankind's needs, and in the center of which grew the mysterious, glittering and all-embracing holy twin to the tree of knowledge, the tree of life itself. In mundane paradise gardens, the place of the tree was taken by a simple shrub or fruit tree, or by a sundial, another symbol of cosmic order and the harmony of the spheres. Paths would wind in labyrinthine, orderly curves among the herbs about this central point, frequently bordered with low, clipped hedges of shrubby herbs or box: ". . . it [the path] may eyther be set with Isope and Time [hyssop and thyme], or with Winter Savery and Time; for these do well endure all ye winter through greene. And there be some which set their mazes with Lavender, Cotton Spike [santolina], Marjerome and such like," advised one sixteenth-century gardening manual.[1] Parkinson, Queen Elizabeth's and King James's own herbalist, on the other hand, advocated a box border, which, he says, "serveth very well to set out any knot or border out any beds, for besides that it is ever greene, it being reasonable thicke set, will easily be cut and formed into any fashion one will." [2] The paths themselves were usually paved with gravel, flagstones, or, in Tudor times, brick. Alternatively they were carpeted with low ground-cover herbs like burnet, creeping thyme, or camomile, each contributing its own special fragrance when trodden underfoot to that of the box or lavender hedge.

Today's herbalist will probably have neither the space, the time, nor the energy, not to say the money, to donate to such horticultural extravagances. "Gardens of memory" and "remberance," "bowers," "mazes," "pleasaunces," and Tudor "knot gardens" are things of the past now for the majority of us. However, a few bricks or steppingstones placed strategically among your herbs are still a good idea for wet weather, and they don't cost that much. If you do decide to grow an herb hedge as a border or windbreak, use rosemary, lavender, germander, santolina, or sage rather than box. Box has an unfortunate tendency to harbor slugs and snails. To combat this perennial menace the old herbalists used to keep toads in their gardens, providing them with little shelters made from tipped-over flowerpots. This happens to be an extremely ecologically sound method of keeping your garden free of pests. But for those who aren't charmed by the idea of pet toads, commercial snail bait will do the job just as well. Keep it away from the herbs themselves, though.

Two last important points: Make sure you plant tall herbs, like mullein, comfrey, and sweet cicely, and shade-loving herbs, like woodruff, toward the back of your garden. Thyme, camomile, chive, and any frequently used kitchen herb should be placed nearer the front, as accessible as possible. Keep any narcotic or witchy herbs, like nightshade, henbane, or hemlock, quite separate from your regular ones. You don't want to confuse the latter with parsley or dill one dark night as you dash out to snip a sprig for supper.

[1] *The Profitable Art of Gardening*, Thomas Hyll, 1579.
[2] *Paradisus in Sole*, John Parkinson, 1629.

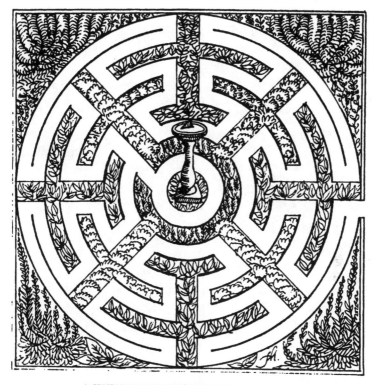

A SEVENTEENTH-CENTURY HERB GARDEN

Finally, if you want to add color to your herb garden, but still keep to "legitimate" herbs, remember that you can always plant jasmine, any type of rose, violets, primroses, foxgloves, lobelia, silvery fringed wormwood, golden thyme, garden valerian, calendula marigolds, and purple basil, and stay within your definition. All these plants are quite properly considered herbs.

INDOOR OR PATIO GARDENS

Herbs take very nicely to pots and containers too, although they do require a little more attention this way. But if you live in a cold climate, it is often best to grow herbs like scented geraniums, lavender, and rosemary in pots anyway. This way you can bring them indoors during really frosty weather.

Any old container will do to grow herbs in, provided it has holes or slits underneath to allow excess water to drain out. Oil cans, barrels, tubs, sitz baths, orange crates—anything can be pressed into service. Scrub the container out well, punch a few holes in the bottom, and make sure it's raised off the ground by a few bricks or a couple of boards to allow for easy drainage. A coat of durable green or white paint on the outside will also do wonders in converting it into an acceptable piece of patio furniture. The flowerpots and planters sold in nurseries are ideal for your purposes. Terracotta strawberry pots make particularly good herb containers: plant your bushier herbs like parsley and sage in the top, and trailers like hanging rosemary, thyme, and marjoram in the little side pockets. Trailing herbs like fringed wormwood and savory also look very handsome in pots suspended by wires, leather thongs, or macramé slings from the ceiling. Only be sure to hang them where the water dripping from their drainage holes won't do any damage. To prevent this you can place your terracotta pot inside a holeless glazed one. Just don't let any water build up inside or the herbs' roots will begin rotting. Similarly, pots placed on a damageable surface like a wooden sideboard can also be set in glazed terracotta saucers.

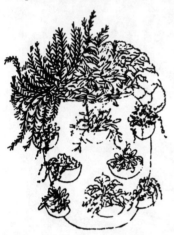

THE LOCATION OF YOUR HERBS

Most potted herbs need on an average half a day's sun. A full day's sun is not really necessary and, in hot climates, not even advisable, as intense heat tends to dry them out too quickly. If you have neither a sunny patio, roof, nor windowsill, never mind: at many nurseries you can buy fluorescent tubes specially made for indoor, sunless horticulture. In any case, the mints, woodruff, sweet cicely, balm, lovage, and chervil, although needing light, grow quite well without direct sun.

If your indoor herbs are planted in pots, rotate them from time to time to allow all sides to get an equal share of the light and prevent the herbs from looking as though they were trying to escape out of the window. Also pinch off the tops every now and then to encourage lateral growth.

TRANSPLANTING HERBS

If you buy your herbs in seedling form from a nursery or mail-order company, transplant them to a larger container as soon as possible. Mix up topsoil from your garden or yard, if you have one, with an equal amount of bark or leaf mold and 1 teaspoon bone meal per 6-inch-diameter pot. Both leaf mold and bone meal are obtainable from your local nursery. If you don't have a yard to obtain topsoil, simply use commercial potting mix, again obtainable from your local nursery or plant store.

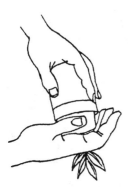

Soak the seedling in its little plastic pot with water. When the excess liquid has drained out, carefully invert the pot, holding one hand over the top and allowing the herb to poke out between your fingers. Tap the plastic until you feel the root ball and earth come loose and rest against your palm. You may find that some of the herb's rootlets have already become entangled in the pot's drainage holes, so you should squeeze the plastic repeatedly with your free hand to encourage them to detach themselves. If you do lose one or two little roots in the process, too bad; it will grow some more. Now transfer the herb gently to its new home, keeping the roots encased in their native soil as much as

possible. Plant it so that the surface of
the root ball comes within 1 inch of the
top of your container. Incidentally, if
you are transferring seedlings you have
raised from seed yourself, transplant
them as soon as they display four obvious leaves. However, check them first
for aphids or red spider mites. If they
do show any signs of bug infestation,
spray them with a mild solution of
yellow naphtha soap and water. Do not
spray poison on any herbs you plan to
use.

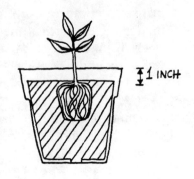

WATERING

A little water every day is the best overall diet for indoor herbs,
especially if you have central heating. One way of telling whether a
pot has dried out is to tap the side and listen to the sound produced.
If it gives a dully heavy clunk, the pot probably still contains water.
If it rings, however, there are air spaces within, and it needs watering.

Watering is best done in the evening. Use a fine spray can
obtainable from any nursery, florist, or hardware store: the type of
plastic spray bottle used for ironing is quite adequate, although
many florists now stock handsome little brass cans especially for the
purpose. Try not to displace the earth or bend the leaves too much
when you spray, although you should make sure all the leaves get a
gentle washing. They contain tiny microscopic vents called stomata
which exhale water-vapor and gases and need to be kept clean. Give
your herbs enough water to ensure that the earth is quite damp.
Another method of ensuring this is to water the herbs from the
bottom, filling the saucers with water and allowing the plant to soak
up as much as it needs through the pot's drainage holes. But in any
case, whether you water from the top or from the bottom, don't
omit the spray.

Once a month you can also treat your herbs to a little fertilizer, either in liquid or in pellet form inserted in the earth. This will ensure good, healthy growth.

TEMPERATURE AND HUMIDITY

If you want to be really serious about growing herbs, keep the temperature of the air around them at about 70° and the humidity level between 30 and 60 per cent. You can check this by means of a hygrometer purchasable at hardware, sports, or craft shops.

TALKING TO THEM

One last point. Don't be afraid to talk to your herbs. Yes, you can wait till no one else is around to listen, but don't omit it. If you want a flourishing herb garden, talk to them at least once a week. If you really cannot manage this for some reason (such as a scoffing skeptical mate), at least discipline yourself to think positive, encouraging, *loud* thoughts to them while you tend them. *Like* your herbs. Plants are very touchy and very sensitive, and enjoy being appreciated. They also sense every mood. Never water them while you're in a rage: it's the surest way to disaster!

PROPAGATION BY CUTTINGS

If you want to take cuttings from your own or a friend's herbs, do this during the spring or summer to allow them warm weather to put down roots. Most of the Labiatae respond well to this type of propagation—balm, hyssop, marjoram, thyme, lavender, rosemary, sage, and so on. Many home gardeners just snap off a twig and shove it in the ground, with perfectly satisfactory results. However, if you want to be more exact, here is the procedure you should follow:

Cut a 3- to 6-inch-long new sprout off the parent plant, snipping it off just below a leaf bud or stem joint. Now place the severed end in a mixture of rooting compound and 2 parts sand and 1 part vermiculite, all obtainable from a nursery. Or simply stick the ends of your cuttings in a jar of water and rooting compound such as Rootone, and leave them to send out threadlike root filaments. It's as easy as that. Soft-stemmed plants like spearmint generally take a week or two to produce roots, woody ones like lavender a month or two.

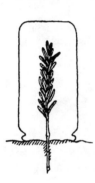

When you come to plant your rooted cuttings, make sure you strip the lower stems of leaves and soak the earth around them well. They need plenty of moisture. You can also place a glass jar, a bell, or even a transparent plastic bag over the cutting to keep the moisture level high. Lift it every other day to allow fresh air in and prevent it from going moldy, though. Also give it plenty of light, but not direct sunlight. (Because of all these conditions, many gardeners start their cuttings indoors.)

PROPAGATION BY LAYERING

An even simpler and surer method of propagation is layering. This means simply that you take one of the still attached branches of the parent herb (the Labiatae respond best to this method) and bend it gently down to the ground. Where it touches the earth, scrape away the leaves and spread the base of the stem with rooting compound. Then bury this loop in the loose soil, allowing the end to poke up into the air. In a month or so you will find that the branch has put down roots through the buried loop; it can then be severed and transplanted to form a new bush.

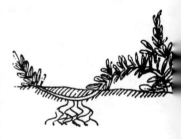

HARVESTING YOUR HERBS

The best time to harvest herbs grown for their flowers or leaves is during the summer. Seeds should be harvested when they appear; roots like dandelion or ginseng in the fall or winter when the leaves have died down.

Early morning after the dew has evaporated is the traditional time for herb gathering. Hyssop, lavender, thyme, and rosemary should be picked when they are in full flower. Sage, on the other hand, should be gathered when the flower buds first appear. Prolific or shrubby herbs like lavender and rosemary can be cut a third of the way down their stems, which, apart from keeping the parent plants healthy and bushy, allows you to dry your crop in bunches hung from the ceiling. Leafy herbs, however, like sorrel, costmary, and fennel, should have only selected leaves plucked from their stems: you don't want to denude them all at once, but rather allow them to continue to produce throughout the year. Chives, parsley, and chervil should be cut just above root level, as they continually send up new shoots. All shrubby perennials, like lavender, marjoram, rosemary, and savory, should in any case be pruned back by at least half the year's growth after they finish flowering to ensure further healthy growth the following year.

DRYING AND STORING

If your harvested herbs are muddy from rain spattering, wash them briefly in cold water when you bring them indoors, and shake off the moisture well. A lettuce shaker is useful here for loose leaves. They can then be patted dry in paper towels.

Any warm, airy room or space can be used for your drying process: a hot-air cupboard, kitchen, dry porch, or furnace room. An unused garage can also serve, provided you don't keep a car in it: exhaust fumes and the smell of gasoline will permeate any herbs you hang up to dry.

Tie long-stemmed herbs and roots in bunches and hang them from nails or a clothesline suspended from wall to wall. You can cover these bunches with paper bags or tissue to prevent dust from gathering on them if you wish. Or else you can cut them into 6-inch stalks and dry them until they are crisp in a 200° oven, being careful that they don't turn brown. Roots can be sliced to facilitate drying if you wish, although ginseng root is best dried whole if you plan to market it.

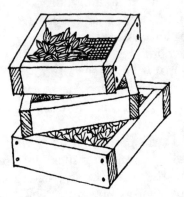

Seeds, small herbs, or individual leaves can be dried in empty shoeboxes or typing-paper boxes. If you're feeling creative you can make effective drying trays out of 1- by 3-inch wood frames backed by fine-mesh window screening. These can be filled with drying herbs and stacked in quite a small space. Failing any of these things, simply lay your herbs out to dry on clean sheets of white lining paper. Once the leaves are crisp, strip them from their stems, leaving them whole if you plan to use them for infusions or poultices, crushing them if you want them for seasonings. Powdered herbs take up less storage space in any event. All leftover dried stems of rosemary, lavender, sage, santolina, southernwood, tansy, thyme, woodruff, and wormwood can now be tied into small aromatic bundles and kept for burning on log fires in winter.

HOW TO PRESERVE FRESH HERBS

Fresh culinary herbs can like roses, be salted in layers and kept in the refrigerator for future use in savory dishes. The salt will also absorb their flavor. Or they may be completely frozen without the addition of salt. This is really about the only way to preserve fresh herbs indefinitely for winter use, especially if they are annuals which die off, like basil or tarragon. Chives, sage, and the mints can also be easily preserved this way. Just wash the freshly picked leaves, pat them dry in paper towels, bag or wrap them in plastic, and throw them in the freezer. Simple.

STORING YOUR HERBS

Keep your dried herbs in airtight opaque or semiopaque containers at an even temperature (e.g., not in a windowsill in the full sun) or they will lose their flavor very quickly. Check them during the first week of packaging to make sure no moisture appears on the inside of the container. If it does, the herb is not sufficiently dry, and should be spread out to crisp for a few more days.

MARKETING YOUR HERBS

If you grow and process a sufficient quantity of an herb and feel like marketing it but don't know where to go, try checking with some of the herb mail-order companies. Those that do not grow their own herbs are sometimes pleased to hear from new sources of fresh herbs. They generally require bulk orders, however, often with minimum orders of, say, 30 pounds, and will always require a sample first.

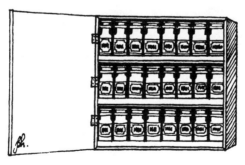

AN HERB CABINET

When you mail your herbs, make sure they are packaged in air- and watertight containers, such as plastic bags or paper wrappings enclosed in tin boxes. Make absolutely sure they are quite dry, too, before you send them. Mildewed herbs are, of course, quite unacceptable.

Finally, if you feel like starting a mail-order herb business of your own, be prepared for a lot of hard work. And buy a book on the subject first. There are all sorts of dodges and shortcuts, not to mention pitfalls, which a beginner should know about. The U.S. government issues a number of useful pamphlets pertaining to mail order, and there are any number of handy books on the market dealing with the subject.

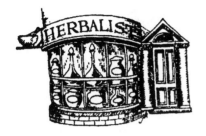

9

WHERE TO BUY YOUR HERBS

TODAY THERE ARE A WIDE RANGE of Internet sites as well as regular mail-order houses that deal specifically in herbs, spices, essential oils, and related matters. Their prices and selections of merchandise vary and it would be impossible to give a complete assessment of the merits of each one. I can only account for those that I know or have used, and I cannot take responsibility for the service the places listed may provide to others. I am also not a qualified medical practitioner nor herbal therapist, so I should not be held responsible for results obtained from the use or misuse of any herbs mentioned in this book or promoted by any of the listed herb sources. Although there is a great deal of promising research currently conducted into the use of herbs and essential oils in the treatment of serious disease and psychological disorders, any reader who is seeking relief from major medical problems is strongly urged to get advice from a qualified medical practitioner before embarking on any program of herbal self-medication.

Those interested in finding an herb source nearby so that they may browse or inspect the merchandise in person should consult their local business telephone directory or the Internet. For me, this

330 / MASTERING HERBALISM

is all part of the enjoyment of herbs—I find herb stores and book-stores hard to resist.

United States

APHRODISIA
264 Bleecker St.
New York, New York 10014

Situated between Sixth and Seventh Avenues, Aphrodisia, in business since the 1970s, offers a range of oils, aromatherapy gear, candles, and herbs, "to jump start your love life," as the store puts it.

CAPRILAND'S HERB FARM
534 Silver St. / Coventry, Connecticut 06328
www.caprilands.com
Phone: (860) 742-7244 / Credit Card Orders: (800) 568-7132

Besides offering lecture programs on herbs and allied subjects, Capriland's carries a wide selection of bulk and freeze-dried herbs, live plants, teas and tisanes, botanicals, oils, fragrances, and potpourris.

FRONTIER NATURAL PRODUCTS CO-OP
www.frontiercoop.com
Phone: (800) 786-1388

Frontier began in Iowa in a small cabin on the Cedar River in 1976 with a very basic line of herbs and spices. Its product line has now grown to ten thousand items, including a wide variety of herbs and spices, spice blends, dried broths and vegetables, potpourris, essential and fragrance oils, organic coffees, herbal and black teas, natural herbal extracts, herb capsules, and homeopathic remedies. A large part of its 77,200 square foot acreage is devoted to growing its herbs, prairie restoration, and a wildlife habitat.

GLENBROOK FARMS HERBS & SUCH
15922 76th St.
Live Oak, Florida 32060
Phone: (888) 716-7627 / Fax: (904) 362-5321

Glenbrook was started in 1996 by Lucinda Jenkins, a retired nurse with a life-long passion for growing herbs and studying their medicinal properties. The company features more than eight hundred bulk herbs and spices, a collection of teas from around the world, essential oils, books, and, interestingly, herbs for horses.

HERB PRODUCTS COMPANY
11012 Magnolia Blvd. / North Hollywood, California 91606
www.herbproducts.com
Phone: (818) 761-0351

Proprietors of botanicals and related herbal products since 1965, Herb Products offers more than five hundred bulk botanicals for preparing teas and capsules, a large assortment of essential and aromatic oils, extracts, and books.

INDIANA BOTANIC GARDENS
P.O. Box 5
Hammond, Indiana 46325
Phone: (800) 644-8327 / Fax: (219) 947-4148

This illustrious company was founded in 1910 by none other than Joseph E. Meyer, the famous American herbalist whose ever-popular book *The Herbalist* is in many ways to the American herbalists what Grieve's *Modern Herbal* is to the English. The company will send on request a booklet about its herbal formulas, nutrients, teas, and other preparations.

LHASA KARNAK HERB COMPANY
2513 Telegraph Ave.
Berkeley, California 94704
Phone: (510) 548-0380

In business since 1970, Lhasa Karnak offers a fine selection of herbs, teas, and essential oils.

MEADOWBROOK HERB GARDEN
93 Kingstown Rd.
Wyoming, Rhode Island 02898

This well-established botanical source offers certified organic seasoning spices, herbs, and herbal teas.

MERRY GARDENS
P.O. Box 595
Camden, Maine 04843
Phone: (207) 236-9064

Like many of the businesses that grow their own produce, Merry
Gardens will send out live seedlings. Although its principle stock
seems to be regular garden plants, it also carries a range of herbs and
scented geraniums.

NICHOLS GARDEN NURSERY
1190 Old Salem Rd. NE / Albany, Oregon 97321-4580
www.nicholsgardennursery.com
Phone: (866) 408-4851

Nichols Garden Nursery has supplied seeds and plants to home and
market gardeners for fifty years through its seventy-two herbs and
rare seed catalog that it now offers online. The owners welcome visitors to their herb gardens to see their herb varities growing. Most
days they will offer visitors a cup of herb tea in the shop, from 8:30
a.m. to 5 p.m. Mondays through Saturdays. They are closed on Sun-
days and major holidays.

PENN HERB COMPANY, LTD
603 N. 2nd St. / Philadelphia, Pennsylvania 19123
www.pennherb.com
Phone: (800) 523-9971

Penn Herb Company, Ltd., a family-owned company, first started
doing business in 1924. It now offers more than seven thousand

herbs, botanicals, natural remedies, essential oils, books, and herb-related items from its own stock. The complete Penn Herb catalog is available online.

HERB BOTTLES AND CONTAINERS

BURCH BOTTLE & PACKING, INC.
811 Tenth St.
Watervliet, New York 12189
Phone: (800) 903-2830

LAVENDER LANE
7337 #1 Roseville Rd.
Sacramento, California 95842
Phone: (888) 593-4400

SUNBURST BOTTLE COMPANY
5710 Auburn Blvd., Suite 7
Sacramento, California 95841
www.sunburstbottle.com

United Kingdom

AQUA OLEUM
Unit 3, Lower Wharf
Wallbridge
Stroud, Gloucestershire GL5 3JA

This is a small family business located in Cotswolds and owned by Alec and Julia Lawless. Julia Lawless is responsible for the highly useful and popular *Encyclopedia of Essential Oils*, and the aim of the company is to provide a selection of the finest essential oils available.

G. BALDWIN & COMPANY
173 Walworth Rd.
London SE17 1RW

Established in 1814, Baldwin carries an extensive range of bulk herbs, essential oils, books, bottles and jars, incenses, and homeopathic and Bach flower remedies.

CULPEPER
Culpeper House
21 Bruton St. / Berkeley Square, London W1X 7DA
Phone / Fax: (020) 7629 4559

Established in 1927, the Bruton Street Culpeper store carries high-quality essential oils, simple herbal remedies, spices, various potpourris, and books. It also has its own brands of assorted natural herbal products, soaps, and cosmetics. There are Culpeper shops in other locations around the country:

LONDON
8 The Piazza / Covent Garden, London WC2E 8HD
Phone / Fax: (020) 7379 6698

BATH
28 Milsom St. / Bath BA1 1DG
Phone / Fax: (012) 2542 5875

BIRMINGHAM
34 The Pavilions, High St. / Birmingham B4 7SL
Phone / Fax: (012) 1643 0100

BOURNEMOUTH
1 Post Office Rd. / Bournemouth BH1 1DN
Phone / Fax: (012) 0255 7107

BRIGHTON
12d Meeting House Ln. / Brighton BN1 1HB
Phone / Fax: (012) 7332 7939

CAMBRIDGE
25 Lion Yard / Cambridge CB2 3NA
Phone / Fax: (012) 2336 7370

CANTERBURY
11 Marlowe Arcade / Canterbury CT1 2PT
Phone / Fax: (012) 2745 1121

CHELTENHAM
17 Pittville St. / Cheltenham GL52 2LN
Phone / Fax: (012) 4257 1784

CHESTER
24 Bridge St. / Chester CH1 1NQ
Phone / Fax: (012) 4431 7774

GUILDFORD
25 Swan Ln. / Guildford GC1 4EQ
Phone / Fax: (014) 8356 0008

LEARNINGTON SPA
2 Royal Priors / Learnington Spa CV32 4XT
Phone / Fax: (019) 2645 0067

LEEDS
30 County Arcade, Victoria Quarter, Queen Victoria St. /
Leeds LS1 6BH
Phone / Fax: (011) 3247 1870

LIVERPOOL
1 Cavern Walks, Mathew St. / Liverpool L2 6RE
Phone / Fax: (015) 1236 5780

NORWICH
5 White Lion St. / Norwich NR2 1QA
Phone / Fax: (016) 0361 9153

OXFORD
7 New Inn Hall St. / Oxford OX1 2DH
Phone / Fax: (018) 6524 9754

SALISBURY
25 The Maltings / Salisbury SP1 2NJ
Phone / Fax: (017) 2232 6159

SHEFFIELD
2 Orchard Square / Sheffield S1 2FB
Phone / Fax: (011) 4276 9788

SOUTHAMPTON
7 Marlands Shopping Centre / Southampton SO14 7SJ
Phone / Fax: (023) 8063 5190

WINDSOR
48 High St. / Windsor SL4 1LR
Phone / Fax: (017) 5362 1488

YORK
43 Low Petergate / York YO1 7HT
Phone / Fax: (019) 0465 1654

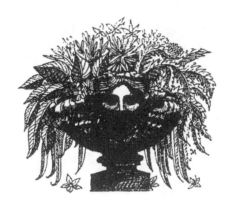

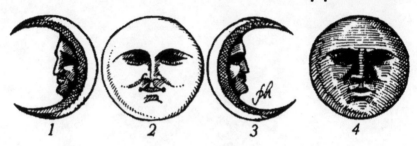

PLANTING AND HARVESTING BY THE MOON

IF YOU WANT TO ADHERE TO THE very oldest traditions of herb growing, you will have to observe the moon's phases for your gardening. According to age-old beliefs still adhered to very conscientiously in many farmers' almanacs, the moon regulates all plant growth. Herbs that yield their harvest aboveground should be sown or planted when the moon is waxing, during its first and second quarters. This includes any leaf, seed, or flower. Root crops such as ginseng, dandelion, and orris, on the other hand, should be planted when the moon is waning, during its third and fourth quarters. The harvesting of any crop should be done at or just after full moon, although authorities tend to differ on exactly how long after. Some say within the third quarter, others say in the last, depending on whether the crop is intended for immediate consumption or storing. If you want to store it, pick it in the last, toward dark of the moon.

Annual herbs: plant during the first or second lunar phase.
Biennial herbs: plant during the third or fourth lunar phase.
Perennial herbs: plant during the third lunar phase.
Cultivation of the ground: during the fourth lunar phase.
Fall planting: during the third lunar phase.

Grafting or making stem cuttings: during the first or second lunar phase, with the moon passing through one of the watery and fertile signs (Cancer, Scorpio, or Pisces; see below).

Harvesting herbs: during the third or fourth lunar phase, with the moon passing through one of the dry and barren signs (Aries, Leo, Sagittarius, Gemini, or Aquarius; see below).

Picking mushrooms of any sort: full moon.

Planting by the Moon's Signs

Many herb growers not only observe the moon's phase to time their planting and harvesting, but also the particular sign of the zodiac through which she is passing. Some signs are considered to be "fruitful" ones, useful for planting in; others "barren," not so good for planting in, but rather useful for harvesting produce meant for storage, or for destroying pests. Which signs the moon is passing through and when can be looked up easily enough in any of the astrological almanacs listed in the bibliography.

The "Characters" of the Signs of the Zodiac

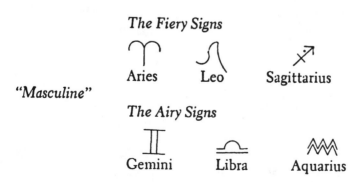

The Fiery Signs

Aries   Leo   Sagittarius

"Masculine"

The Airy Signs

Gemini   Libra   Aquarius

The Watery Signs

♋ Cancer   ♓ Pisces   ♏ Scorpio

"Feminine"

The Earthy Signs

♉ Taurus   ♍ Virgo   ♑ Capricorn

Moon in Aries: Fiery and masculine; dry and barren. Used for
☽ in ♈ cultivating the ground and destroying pests and weeds. Good for gathering all herbs and roots.

Moon in Taurus: Earthy and feminine; moist and fertile. Used for
☽ in ♉ planting any herbs, especially roots, such as ginseng and dandelion.

Moon in Gemini: Airy and masculine; dry and barren. Like Aries,
☽ in ♊ used for cultivation and destroying weeds and pests. Good for gathering all herbs and roots.

Moon in Cancer: Watery and feminine; moist and fertile. Ideal for
☽ in ♋ planting any herb, and also good for irrigation.

Moon in Leo: Fiery and masculine; dry and barren. Again, useful for
☽ in ♌ cultivation, pest or weed control, and gathering all herbs and roots.

Moon in Virgo: Earthy and feminine; moist and barren. Useful for
☽ in ♍ cultivation and pest or weed control only, although you can plant irises now.

Moon in Libra: Airy and masculine; moist and semifertile. Used for
☽ in ♎ planting flowers, vines, and root crops only.

Moon in Scorpio: Watery and feminine; moist and fertile. Almost
☽ in ♏ as productive as Cancer, and especially useful for vines, such as the hop. A good sign to plant any herbs in.

Moon in Sagittarius: Fiery and masculine; dry and barren. Useful
☽ in ♐ for the cultivation of soil and the planting of leeks, onions, or garlic. Good for gathering any herbs.

Moon in Capricorn: Earthy and feminine; dry and fertile. Good for
☽ in ♑ planting roots and rhizomes, such as ginseng and iris.

Moon in Aquarius: Airy and masculine; dry and barren. Good for
☽ in ♒ pest and weed control, ground cultivation, and
gathering all herbs and roots.

Moon in Pisces: Watery and feminine; moist and fertile. Useful for
☽ in ♓ planting any herb, especially where root growth is
required.

WEIGHTS AND MEASURES

Handy Kitchen equivalents

1 minim (liquid measure) = 1 drop
1 grain (dry measure) = 1 drop
1 dram (liquid or dry measure) = 1 teaspoon
2 drams = 1 dessertspoon
½ ounce = 1 tablespoon
1 ounce = 2 tablespoons
2 ounces = 1 wineglass
4 ounces = 1 teacup
8 ounces (dry measure) = 1 (kitchen) cup
2 gills (liquid measure) = 1 (kitchen) cup
1 pound (16 ounces, dry measure) = 2 (kitchen) cups
1 pint (liquid measure) = 2 (kitchen) cups

Official Weights and Measures

(Originally the word "drachm," the old Greek coin "drachma" of
Dioscorides' day, was used in the apothecaries' weights to distin-

guish it from the "dram" of the avoirdupois scale. Nowadays both are confusingly written "dram." Wherever "dram" is referred to in the text, the apothecary weight is meant.)

APOTHECARIES' WEIGHT *(small amounts used in medicine)*

        20 grains = 1 scruple
        3 scruples = 60 minims (liquid) = 1 dram (drachm)
        8 drams = 1 ounce

AVOIRDUPOIS WEIGHT *(larger amounts used in cookery)*

        16 ounces = 1 pound

LIQUID AND DRY MEASURE *(used in beer- and winemaking)*

4 gills = 1 pint (20 ounces avoirdupois of water)
2 pints = 1 quart
2 quarts = 1 pottle
4 quarts = 1 gallon (10 pounds avoirdupois of water)
2 gallons = 1 peck
4 pecks = 1 bushel
8 bushels = 1 quarter
5 quarters = 1 load or wey

2 weys = 1 last
9 gallons = 1 firkin
2 firkins = 1 kilderkin
4 firkins (36 gallons) = 1 barrel
54 gallons = 1 hogshead of ale
63 gallons = 1 hogshead of wine
84 gallons = 1 puncheon
126 gallons = 1 butt or pipe
2 pipes (252 gallons) = 1 tun

Continental European Weights and Measures

LIQUID MEASURES

1 liter = 4½ cups
1 demiliter (½ liter) = 2 (generous) cups
1 deciliter (1/10 liter) = ½ (scant) cup

WEIGHT

1 gram = .035 ounces
28.35 grams = 1 ounce
100 grams = 3½ ounces
114 grams = 4 ounces (approximately)
226.78 grams = 8 ounces
500 grams = 1 pound 1½ ounces (approximately)
1 kilogram (1000 grams) = 2.21 pounds

HERBS
AS NUTRITIONAL SOURCES

VITAMIN A. Alfalfa. Dandelion. Okra.

VITAMIN B_1. Bladderwrack. Fenugreek. Okra. Wheat germ.

VITAMIN B_2. Bladderwrack. Fenugreek. Saffron.

VITAMIN B_{12}. Alfalfa. Bladderwrack.

VITAMIN C. Burdock seed. Calendula. Capsicum. Coltsfoot. Elderberries. Orégano. Paprika. Parsley. Rose hips. Watercress.

VITAMIN D. Watercress. Wheat germ.

VITAMIN E. Alfalfa. Bladderwrack. Dandelion leaves. Linseed. Sesame. Watercress. Wheat germ.

VITAMIN K. Alfalfa. Chestnut leaves. Shepherd's purse.

NIACIN. Alfalfa leaves. Blueberry leaves. Burdock seed. Fenugreek. Parsley. Watercress. Wheat germ.

RUTIN. Buckwheat. Rue. Paprika.

CALCIUM. Arrowroot. Camomile. Chives. Coltsfoot. Dandelion root. Meadowsweet. Nettle. Okra pods. Pimpernel. Plantain. Shepherd's purse. Sorrel.

IODINE. Bladderwrack.

IRON. Burdock root. Meadowsweet. Mullein. Nettle. Parsley. Salep. Strawberry leaves. Watercress.

MAGNESIUM. Bladderwrack. Carrot tops. Dandelion. Kale. Meadowsweet. Mullein. Okra. Parsley. Peppermint. Primrose. Walnut leaves. Watercress. Wintergreen.

PHOSPHORUS. Calamus. Calendula flowers. Caraway seeds. Chickweed. Garlic. Licorice root. Meadowsweet. Okra pods. Sesame. Sorrel. Watercress.

POTASSIUM. Birch bark. Borage. Calamus. Carrot tops. Camomile. Coltsfoot. Comfrey. Dandelion. Eyebright. Fennel. Mullein. Nettle. Parsley. Peppermint. Plantain. Primrose flowers. Savory. Walnut leaves. Watercress. Yarrow.

SODIUM. Chives. Fennel seed. Meadowsweet. Nettle. Okra pods. Shepherd's purse. Sorrel. Watercress.

SULPHUR. Asafoetida. Calamus. Coltsfoot. Eyebright. Fennel seed. Garlic. Meadowsweet. Mullein. Nettle. Okra. Pimpernel. Plantain leaves. Shepherd's purse. Watercress.

A CHRISTIANIZED CONJURATION OF THE HERB VALERIAN

FIRST KNEEL DOWN ON BOTH your knees, your face to the east, and make a cross over the herb, and say, "In the name of the Father, and of the Son, and of the Holy Ghost. Amen."

Then say a Pater Noster, Ave Maria and Creed, also a St. John's Gospel. This must be done secretly, alone on the Friday or Thursday, the Moon being at the full and before you speak a word to any creature. Also you must say before you take him from out of the ground, "I conjure thee herb that are called valerian, for thou art worthy for all things in the world. In pleasance, in Court before Kings, Rulers, and Judges thou makest friendship so great that they bare thee his will, for thou doest great miracles. The ghosts of Hell do bow to thee and obey thee. For whosoever hath thee, whatsoever he desireth, he shall have in the name of the Father, of the Son and of the Holy Ghost. Amen."

Keep it cleane in a faire cloth.

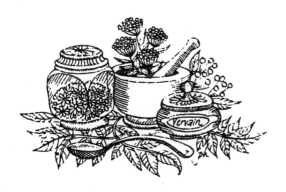

GLOSSARY

ACTIVE. Adjective applied to a medicinally potent herb in a blend.

AGENT. A perfumery term indicating the dominant fragrance in a blend.

ALCOHOL. A liquid obtained by distilling fermented organic liquors. Only alcohol sold for culinary purposes should be used in edible or potable herbal preparations. *Never* use household alcohol or wood alcohol. If you cannot obtain potable wine alcohol (also known as ethyl alcohol or wine spirit), a regular commercial spirit such as brandy, whiskey, gin, or vodka may be used instead. For colognes and preparations intended for external application only, medicinal alcohol (95 or 84 per cent) may be used.

ALKALOID. A vegetable substance with an organic nitrogen base capable of combining with acids to form an easily assimilable crystalline salt. Alkaloids exert a powerful influence over an organism even when ingested in small amounts. Chemical alkaloids all end in *-ine* (e.g., harmaline, the drug obtained from rue). Those organic chemicals that end in *-in*, e.g., digitalin (foxglove) have a similar powerful action, but do not react with acids.

ALTERATIVE. An herb given by herbalists to mildly purge the system; often a blood purifier or a simple nutrient.

ALTERNATE. Botanical term meaning placed on opposite sides of the stem on different levels.

ANALGESIC. A pain-killing herb.

ANAPHRODISIAC. An herb that lessens sexual inclination or function.

ANNUAL. Botanical term meaning a plant that lasts only a single year or season.

ANODYNE. A pain-killing herb.

ANTHELMINTIC. An herb which expels or destroys worms.

ANTISCORBUTIC. An herb that acts as a preventative of scurvy, a diseased condition of the blood arising from vitamin C deficiency.

347

ANTISEPTIC. An herb that inhibits the growth of bacteria on living tissue.

ANTISPASMODIC. An herb that allays convulsions or muscular spasms.

APERIENT. A laxative herb.

APHRODISIAC. An herb that increases sexual inclination or function.

APOTHECARY. An old term for a person who prepares and sells medicines.

AROMATIC. A fragrant herb or spice possessing mildly stimulating properties.

ASTRINGENT. An herb that causes the contraction of tissues.

AXIL. A botanical term referring to the hollow where the base of a leaf joins its stem.

BALM. 1. A common name for the herb *Melissa officinalis.* 2. An old variation of the word "balsam" (q.v.).

BALSAM. 1. The fragrant gum or sap of a plant or tree. 2. A soothing ointment.

BIENNIAL. A botanical term referring to a plant that takes two years to reach maturity.

BLENDER. A perfumery term referring to a secondary fragrance in a perfume blend.

BOTANY. The scientific study of plants.

CALYX. A botanical term referring to the outer "cup" or whorl (q.v.) of petals or leaves on a flower.

CARMINATIVE. An herb or spice that expels wind from the stomach and intestines.

CATHARTIC. A laxative herb.

CORDIAL. A stimulating beverage.

CULL, TO. An old herbal term meaning to pick or pluck.

DECIDUOUS. A botanical term referring to trees or plants that lose their leaves in the winter.

DECOCTION. An herbal preparation made by boiling an herb, generally a bark, root, or seed, in a covered enamel or other wise nonmetallic container of water for 15 minutes or longer.

DEMONOFUGE. An old term for an herb thought to expel evil spirits.

DEMULCENT. An herb which, when ingested, lubricates and coats the stomach and intestine linings.

DENTATE. A botanical term referring to a notched or indented leaf edge.

DIAPHORETIC. A perspiration-promoting herb. Also known as a sudorific.

DIGESTIVE; DIGESTANT. An herb that aids the digestion.

DISTILL, TO. To extract an herbal essence by a process of boiling the herb in a liquid and condensing the vapor that arises.

DIURETIC. An herb that stimulates kidney action and encourages the discharge of urine.

ELIXIR. A distillation or tincture (q.v.).

EMETIC. An herb with the power to cause vomiting.

EMMENAGOGUE. An herb that promotes menstruation.

EMOLLIENT. An herb used externally for its soothing, softening properties.

ENFLEURAGE. A perfumery term referring to the production of perfume by soaking flower petals in oil or alcohol.

ESSENCE. 1. A solution, often comprising a mixture of water and alcohol, obtained from herbs either by decoction or distillation. 2. 1 ounce essential oil dissolved in 1 pint alcohol.

ESSENTIAL OIL. Quickly evaporating and odoriferous oil produced in the seeds, flowers, leaves, stems, and roots of many herbs.

EVERGREEN. A botanical term referring to a plant or tree that keeps its leaves throughout the winter.

EXPECTORANT. An herb which helps to loosen and expel catarrh.

EXTRACT. A strong decoction.

FEBRIFUGE. An herb which helps to dispel fever.

FIXATIVE. A perfumery term referring to a substance added to a perfume blend to absorb and preserve more fugitive scents.

FLORET. A botanical term referring to a single small flower from a cluster.

GENUS (plural: genera). A Latin botanical term meaning a plant family.

HABITAT. A Latin botanical term referring to the location where a wild herb may be found.

HALLUCINOGEN. A drug that produces hallucinations.

HERBAL. A book of herb lore.

HERBALISM. The study of herbs as performed by an herbalist.

HERBARIST. A person who grows or sells herbs.

HERBARY. A medieval herb garden.

HIPPOCRAS. A spiced wine beverage.

HIPPOCRATES SLEEVE. A fine net for straining herbal brews.

HOMEOPATHY. The belief that diseases can be cured by minute amounts of certain herbally derived drugs which in a healthy person produce symptoms similar to those exhibited by the patient.

HYDROMEL. A honey drink.

INFUSION. A strong herbal tea.

LATERAL. A botanical term meaning branching on either side of the stem.

LAXATIVE. An herb which loosens the bowels. Also called an aperient.

LEECH. An Anglo-Saxon word for a healer. The art of the leech is leechcraft or leechdom.

LEECHBOOK. An Anglo-Saxon book of medicine.

LINEAR. A botanical term meaning narrow or slender.

LOBE. A botanical term meaning a round division of a leaf.

LOTION. A liquid herbal preparation for external use.

MACERATE, TO. To soak an herb, generally in oil or alcohol.

MEAD. An archaic drink made from honey and herbs.

MUCILAGE. Natural gum derived from plants.

MULCH. A surface layer of rotted leaves or manure spread on the ground to keep the roots of plants moist or warm.

NARCOTIC. Causing sleep or coma.

NERVINE. A tonic herb that strengthens the nerves.

OPPOSITE. A botanical term referring to leaves arranged in pairs on either side of the stem.

PERENNIAL. A botanical term meaning a plant which lives for more than two years.

PESTLE. A blunt instrument used to crush and grind herbs. Its bowl-shaped complementary container is known as a mortar. Most kitchenware stores sell these today.

PHARMACOPOEIA. A list of drugs and formulas.

PHILTER, TO. To strain an herbal beverage.

PISTIL. The ovary-bearing female organ of a flower.

POSSET. A drink made from hot milk curdled with ale or wine.

POTION. An herbal drink.

POTPOURRI. A fragrant blend of herbs, spices and oils used to perfume the house.

POULTICE. A warm, damp pack of herbs applied to a wound or sprain to draw the blood and relieve pain.

PSYCHOACTIVE. A consciousness-altering herb, often hallucinogenic (q.v.) or narcotic (q.v.).

PURGATIVE. Laxative.

REFRIGERANT. An herb that cools the blood, or appears to do so.

RHIZOME. A botanical term meaning a horizontal, thickened, rootlike stem, from which spring small rootlets. Orris root is a rhizome.

RUBIFACIENT. An herb which produces redness of the skin.

SACHET. A small cloth bag of herbs or spices.

SACK. An old term for white wine.

SEARCE, TO. To sift.

SEDATIVE. An herb that calms or tranquilizes.

SERRATED. A botanical term referring to a leaf edge notched like a saw.

SIMPLE. A single herb given as a remedy.

SOLUTION. A substance that has been combined with a liquid.

SPATULATE. A botanical term meaning "spreading" or "trowel-shaped."

STAMEN. The pollen-bearing male organ of a flower.

STILL-ROOM BOOK. An eighteenth-century privately kept book of herbal recipes.

STIMULANT. An herb that quickens some vital process.

STOMACHIC. An herb that aids the stomach.

STYPTIC. A blood-staunching herb.

SUFFUMIGATION. 1. An application of smoke or fumes. 2. Incense.

SYRUP. 1. A mixture of herbal extract and sugar. 2. A bottled infusion sealed from the air by the addition of glycerin.

TINCTURE. A mixture of herbal extract and alcohol. One to 4 ounces powdered herb added to 4 ounces water and 12 ounces alcohol left to stand for 14 davs before filtering will produce a tincture. A layer of glycerin is often floated on top to aid preservation.

TISANE. A French word for an herb tea.

TONIC. 1. An herb that stimulates some part of the body. 2. An herb that provides nutrition to some part of the body.

TRITURATION. A process of rubbing herbs and spices down to a fine powder and blending them.

UNGUENT. An archaic term for ointment or salve. Herbal unguents may be made with 8 parts heated lanolin, beeswax and olive oil, Vaseline, lard or other fatty medium, into which is mixed 2 parts finely powdered herbs. Another old method is to boil herbs in water until a strong extract is formed, strain it, then add it to warm (not hot) olive oil. Bring it to a boil, and simmer until the water has completely evaporated, leaving only the oil. Now add enough beeswax and rosin to solidify the ointment, stirring continuously.

VARIEGATED. A botanical term meaning formed from or patched with an assortment of colors.

VERMIFUGE. Worm expellant.

VOLATILE. Quickly evaporating.

VULNERARY. Styptic (q.v.) and often antiseptic. Literally, "wound-healing."

WHORL. A circular set of leaves or petals surrounding a stem.

WORT. An Anglo-Saxon word for an herb.

WORTCUNNING. Anglo-Saxon for herb lore.

SELECT BIBLIOGRAPHY

THE OLD HERBALISTS

Apuleius, *Herbarium.* M. S. Harleian 5294, British Museum.

Banckes, Richard, *Bankes's Herbal.* 1525.

Coles, William, *Adam in Eden, or Nature's Paradise.* London, 1657.

———, *The Art of Simpling.* London, 1656.

Culpeper, Nicholas, *The English Physician Or an Astrologo-physical Discourse of the Vulgar Herbs of this Nation* ... 1652, 1820. Also reprinted by Foulsham, London, as *Culpeper's Complete Herbal* (N.D.).

Gerard, John, *The Herball, or Generall Historie of Plantes.* London, 1597.

———, *Leaves from Gerard's Herball.* Arranged by Marcus Woodward, New York, Dover, 1969.

Goodyer, John (trans.), *The Greek Herbal of Dioscorides.* 1655, ed. Robert T. Gunther, 1933; New York, Hafner, 1968.

Hyll, Thomas, *The Proffitable Arte of Gardeninge.* 1568.

Leechbook of Bald and Cild, The. M. S. Royal 12 D., British Museum.

Macer, Aemilius, *Of the virtues of herbs.* English trans. M. S. Sloane 140, British Museum.

Parkinson, John, *Paradisi in Sole Paradisus Terrestris.* London, 1629.

———, *Theatrum Botanicum.* London, 1640.

Pliny the Elder, *Natural History.* Loeb Classical Library.

Ram, William, *Ram's Little Dodoen.* London, 1606.

Turner, William, *A new Herball.* London, 1551.

Tusser, Thomas, *Five Hundred Pointes of Good Husbandrie,* London, 1573.

352

HERBAL MEDICINES AND FORMULAS

Culbreth, D., *Materia Medica.* Philadelphia, Lea & Febiger, 1927.
Fernie, Dr., *Herbal Simples.* 1897.
Grieve, Mrs. M., *A Modern Herbal.* 2 vols., New York, Hafner Publishing, 1967, 1970.
Harris, Ben Charles, *The Compleat Herbal.* Barre, Massachusetts, Barre Publishers, 1972.
Lucas, Richard, *Common and Uncommon Uses of Herbs for Healthful Living.* New York, Arco Publishing Co., N.D.
———, *The Magic of Herbs in Daily Living.* New York, Parker Publishing, 1972.
———, *Nature's Medicines.* New York, Parker Publishing, 1966.
Meyer, Joseph E., *The Herbalist.* 1918; revised editions, 1960, 1970 (obtainable through Indiana Botanic Gardens).
National Formulary. 13th edition, American Pharmaceutical Association, Mack Publishing, 1970.
Rose, Jeanne, *Herbs and Things.* New York, Grosset & Dunlap, 1972.

HERB COOKERY AND HOUSEHOLD RECIPES

Dawson, T., *The Good Housewife's Jewell.* 1586.
Digby, Sir Kenelm, *Choice and Experimental Receipts.* 1668.
———, *The Closet of Sir Kenelm Digby Opened.* 1669.
Doggett, Mary, *Mary Doggett: Her Book of Receipts.* 1682.
Evelyn, J., *Acetaria: A Book about Sallets.* 1680.
Grieve, Mrs. M., *Culinary Herbs and Condiments.* New York, Harcourt, Brace, 1934.
Larousse Gastronomique. New York, Crown, 1961.
Platt, Sir Hugh, *Delights for Ladies.* 1594.
Rohde, Eleanour Sinclair, *A Garden of Herbs.* London, the Medici Society, 1921; New York, Dover, 1969.
Smith, E., *The Compleat Housewife.* 1736.
Sounin, Leonie de, *Magic in Herbs.* New York, Pyramid Books, 1972.

NARCOTIC AND HALLUCINOGENIC HERBS

De Ropp, R. S., *Drugs and the Mind.* New York, Grove Press, 1957.
Eliade, Mircea, *Shamanism: Archaic Techniques of Ecstasy.* New York, Pantheon, 1964.
Emboden, William A., *Narcotic Plants.* New York, Macmillan, 1972.
Harner, Michael J. (ed.), *Hallucinogens and Shamanism.* New York, Oxford University Press, 1973.
Lewin, Louis, *Phantastica, Narcotic and Stimulating Drugs: Their Use and Abuse.* New York, E. P. Dutton, 1964.
Superweed, M. J., *Herbal Highs.* San Francisco, Stone Kingdom Syndicate, 1970.

HERBAL APHRODISIACS

Davenport, John, *Aphrodisiacs and Anti-aphrodisiacs.* London, 1869; New York, Award Books, 1970.
Knight, R. P., and Wright, T., *Sexual Symbolism.* New York, Bell Publishing Co., 1957.
Petronius, Caius, *The Satyricon.*
Superweed, M. J., *Herbal Aphrodisiacs.* San Francisco, Stone Kingdom Syndicate, 1971.
Wedeck, H. E., *Love Potions Through the Ages.* New York, Philosophical Library, 1963.

WITCHCRAFT AND WORTCUNNING

Albertus Magnus, *The Egyptian Secrets of Albertus Magnus.* N.P., N.D.
Backster, Cleve, "Evidence of a Primary Perception in Plant Life," *International Journal of Parapsychology,* Vol. 10, No. 4, New York, 1968.
Barrett, Francis, *The Magus.* London, 1801.
Burland, C. A., *The Magical Arts.* London, Arthur Barker, 1966.

Cockayne, O., *Leechdoms, Wortcunning and Starcraft in Early England.* 3 vols., London, 1864–66.

Devore, Nicholas, *Encyclopedia of Astrology.* New York, Philosophical Library, 1947.

Eliade, Mircea, *Patterns in Comparative Religion.* Trans. Rosemary Sheed, New York, Sheed and Ward, 1958.

Frazer, Sir James G., *The Golden Bough.* London, Macmillan and Co., 1922.

Graves, Robert, *The White Goddess.* London, Faber and Faber, 1961.

Grimm, Jacob, *Teutonic Mythology* (1883–88). 4 vols., trans. J. S. Stallybrass; New York, Dover, 1966.

Hohman, J. G., *Pow-wows or, The Long Lost Friend.* Hackensack, New Jersey, Wehman Bros., 1820.

Huson, Paul, *The Devil's Picturebook.* New York, G. P. Putnam's Sons, 1971.

———, *Mastering Witchcraft.* New York, G. P. Putnam's Sons, 1970.

Jacob, Dorothy, *A Witch's Guide to Gardening.* New York, Taplinger, 1964.

Lacnunga—Liber medicinalis de virtutibus herbarum. Ms. Harleian 585, British Museum.

Leland, C. G., *Etruscan Magic and Occult Remedies.* New York, University Books, 1963.

———, *Gipsy Sorcery and Fortune-telling.* New York, University Books, 1963.

Mathers, S. L. M. (trans. and ed.), *The Greater Key of Solomon.* Chicago, De Laurence, Scott & Co., 1914.

Porta, Giovanni Battista (Johannes Baptista), *Natural Magick.* Reproduction of 1658 English text, New York, Basic Books, 1957.

Randolph, Vance, *Ozark Superstitions.* New York, Dover, 1964.

Shah, Sayed Idries, *The Secret Lore of Magic.* Containing *Of the Vertues of Hearbes* by Albertus Magnus, New York, Citadel, 1970.

Singer, Dr. Charles, "Early English Magic and Medicine," in *Proceedings of the British Academy,* vol. IV.

Spence, Lewis, *The Magic Arts in Celtic Britain.* London, Rider, 1946, 1970.

———, *The Mysteries of Britain.* London, Rider, 1928, 1970.

Thompson, C. J. S., *The Mysteries and Secrets of Magic.* London, Bodley Head, 1927.

———, *The Mystic Mandrake.* New York, University Books.

Thorndike, Lynn, *A History of Magic and Experimental Science.* 8 vols., New York, Columbia University Press, 1923–58.

Waite, Arthur Edward, *The Book of Ceremonial Magic*. New York, University Books, 1961.
Walker, D. P., *Spiritual and Demonic Magic from Ficino to Campanella*. London, The Warburg Institute, 1958.

PLANTING BY THE MOON

Harley, Rev. T. H., *Moon Lore*. Rutland, Vermont, and Tokyo, Charles E. Tuttle, 1970.
Herbalist Almanac, The. Indiana Botanic Gardens, Hammond, Indiana 46325. Published annually.
Moon Sign Book, The. Llewellyn Publications, Saint Paul, Minnesota 55101. Published annually.
Old Farmer's Almanac, The. Dublin, N.H. 03444. Published annually.
Raphael's Almanac. W. Foulsham and Co. Ltd., Yeovil Road, Slough, Bucks, England. Published annually.
Witches' Almanac, The. New York, Grosset & Dunlap, RD 2, Box 200, Pine Bush, New York 12566. Published annually.

GINSENG AND ELIXIRS OF LIFE

Eliade, Mircea, *The Forge and the Crucible*. Trans. Stephen Corin, New York, Harper Torchbooks, 1971.
Holmyard, E. J., *Alchemy*. London, Penguin Books, 1957, 1968.
Wallnöfer, H., and Rottauscher, A. V., *Chinese Folk Medicine*. New York, Bell Publishing, 1965.
Williams, Llewelyn, *Growing Ginseng*. U. S. Department of Agriculture Farmers' Bulletin No. 2201, U.S. Government Printing Office, Washington, D.C. 20402.
(See also Lucas, R., *Natures Medicines*; and Lucas, R., *The Magic of Herbs*, op. cit.; Meyer's *Herbalist*, op. cit.; and Grieve's *Modern Herbal*, op. cit.)

HERBS IN GENERAL

Coon, Nelson, *Using Wayside Plants*. New York, Hearthside Press, 1960.

How to Grow Herbs. Menlo Park, California, Lane Books, 1972.

Leyel, C. F., *The Magic of Herbs*. London, Jonathan Cape, 1920.

McCleod, Dawn, *Herb Handbook*. California, Wilshire Book Company, 1968.

Millspaugh, C. F., *American Medicinal Plants*. New York, Boericke & Tafel, 1887.

Novak, F. A., *The Pictorial Encyclopedia of Plants and Flowers*. London, Paul Hamlyn, 1966.

Ranson, F., *British Herbs*. London, Penguin Books, 1954.

Rohde, Eleanour Sinclair, *The Old English Herbals*. London, Longmans, Green, 1922.

Singer, Dr. Charles, *From Magic to Science*. New York, Dover Publications, 1958.

Weiner, Michael A., *Earth Medicine: Earth Foods, Plant Remedies, Drugs, and Natural Foods of the North American Indians*. New York, Collier Books, 1972.

MAIL-ORDER BUSINESS

How to Win Success in the Mail Order Business. New York, Arco Publishing Co., 1966.

INDEX

359